A Complement Work of Present
Acupuncture and Moxibustion

Techniques of
Acupuncture & Moxibustion

Editors-in-chief	*Liu Gongwang*
Translator-in-chief	*Liu Changlin*
English Editor	*Donald P. Lauda*
Translation Revisor	*Liu Gongwang*

HUAXIA PUBLISHING HOUSE

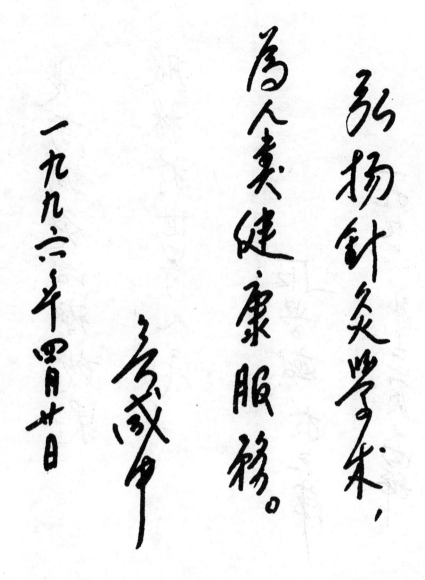

Promote and develop the academic learning of   acupuncture and moxibustion and give service to the   health of humanity!

Wu Xianzhong

April 20，1996

(Inscription by Prof. Wu Xianzhong，Academician of Academy of Engineering of China，Chairman of the Chinese Association of the Integration of Traditional and Western Medicine)

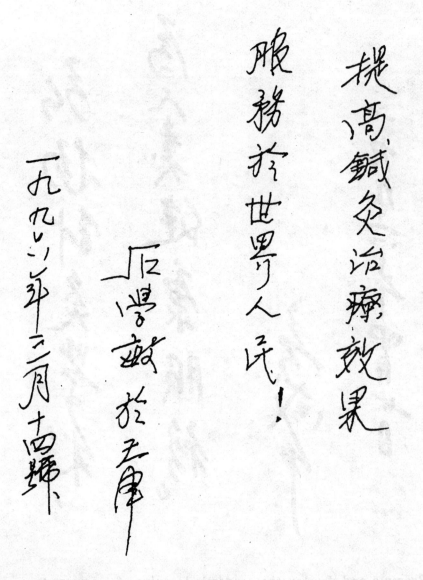

提高鍼灸治療效果
服務於世界人民！

石學敏於天津

一九九六年三月十四號

**Enhance the curative effect of acupuncture-moxibustion thera-
py and serve the people of the world!**

Shi Xuemin

March 14, 1996

(Inscription by Prof. Shi Xuemin, Member of the Council of China
Acupuncture Association, President of the First Hospital Affiliated to
Tianjin College of TCM)

Preface

In the study of acupuncture and moxibustion, command of the techniques of needling and moxibustion is indispensible for beginners. The basis for the right selection of acupoints and their correct manipulation has a direct bearing on the curative effect in clinical practice. Rich experience was accumulated by physicians in successive dynasties during the course of their clinical practice. This laid the foundation for the development of acupuncture and moxibustion

Acupuncture and moxibustion both belong to external treatment as expressed in the book *Plain Questions*（素问，Su Wen）"Sagital stone needle and mugwort moxibustion are used externally". Since the acupuncture appliance used in old times was a kind of stone（named Bian Shi 砭石）,this kind of treatment was also called stone-acupuncture in ancient China. As society progressed, this kind of stone was gradually replaced by different kinds of needles,thus, treatment with them were often called needle-acupuncture,or needling for short. What was called "needle acupuncture" was actually the application of different kinds of needling appliances（mainly the filiform needles) to activate and regulate the meridian-qi by stimulating certain parts（needling points) of the body so as to achieve the purpose of regulating body functions and curing diseases.

Acupuncture may date back to the Neolithic Age. The first surgical appliances in ancient China were sharp cones or cuneiform stones. At first,these stones were only used to tap certain parts of the body, puncturing an area for blood-letting or cutting it to evacuate pus. During their long practice, people discovered and created the stone treatment,which is the predecessor of modern acupuncture.

In addition to cuneiform stones,bone and bamboo were also used as materials to make needles in ancient times. With the invention of alchemy,metal needles gradually replaced stone,bone and bamboo needles. Bronze,iron,gold,silver copper-nickel and alloy needles also appeared. The most commonly used needle at present is the filiform needle which is made of stainless steel alloy. Other needles often used today include the three-edged needle,the skin needle（plum-blossom needle and seven-star needle), the intradermal needle and the scorched needle.

The exposition of nine types of needling in the *Internal Classic*（内经,Nei Jing)

laid a theoretical foundation for acupuncture therapy. Physicians in later ages, guided by the *Internal Classic*(内经, Nei Jing) and the *Classic of Medical Problems*(难经, Nan Jing), created many other needling methods, especially during the Yuan and Ming dynasties. Experiences with acupuncture were published consecutively and acupuncture treatment has developed rapidly ever since.

Moxibustion is a therapy in which ignited mugwort floss, or other medicinal herbs are applied over the affected part of the body. By warming or scorching the affected part, diseases can be prevented and cured. Though acupuncture and moxibustion are two different types of treatment, both are based on the principle of stimulating a specific region and regulating Ying, Wei, Qi and Blood of the human body to treat diseases, thus they are often combined and called "acupuncture and moxibustion".

Moxibustion had its origin in primitive society in China, evolving at a time when people began to use fire. When people made fire to warm themselves, certain parts of their body were accidentally burned or scorched, which surprisingly relieved or even cured certain diseases. From these experiences, people understood that burning or warming certain areas of their bodies could treat diseases. The material used as fuel in moxibustion at first was probably common plant leaves. Later mugwort floss was specifically used, which was clearly recorded in the documents of the Warring States (475— 221 BC). For instance, Mengzi(孟子)said "Patient with a seven-year course of disease must be treated with moxa plant preserved for three years." The application of moxa floss relates closely to its specific properties. It is combustible and its heat permeability is both intense and persistent. It is also cheap and easy to obtain. In ancient times, direct moxibustion was usually administered by applying the burning moxa floss directly on the skin around an acupuncture point. Later, various types of indirect moxibustion were gradually developed, which were conducted by purposely placing something between the burned floss and the acupoint in order to relieve the pain due to the intense heat of direct moxibustion. This would strengthen the therapeutic efficacy by enlarging its treatment scope. A variety of materials were used for separation in indirect moxibustion. The most common were ginger, garlic, salt, prepared aconite root, etc. Now, there are over 40 kinds of materials which can be applied in indirect moxibustion and most of these are medicinal herbs.

Apart from moxibustion with mugwort floss, there are many other forms of moxibustion such as burning rush moxibustion, moxibustion with mulberry twig, electrothermic moxibustion, vapor moxibustion, moxibustion with garlic, moxibustion with mylabris and moxibustion with white mustard seed. But at the present time they are not used often in clinical settings.

In addition to acupuncture and moxibustion, there is another commonly used external treatment called cupping. In ancient times it was called horn cupping, since the appliance used in this therapy was an animal horn. Cupping therapy involves the application of a cup in which a partial vacuum is created by burning something inside the cup over an acupoint. This brings about local congestion and blood stasis, thus attaining the purpose of treating diseases. The first known tool used for cupping was an animal horn. It then evolved from the horn to a pottery cup to a bamboo cup, to a copper cup and to the present day glass cup. The methods of creating a vacuum are by burning, boiling or by pumping. Single-cupping, multiple-cupping, retaining cupping, successive flash-cupping, movable cupping, medicinal cupping and acupuncture cupping are different forms of cupping used today.

Liu Gongwang

1997. 10. 10

English Editor Preface

It has been my personal and professional privilege to serve as the English editor for this book on acupuncture and moxibustion. I feel honored to have had the opportunity to review the work of such distinguished and knowledgeable individuals. This book continues the rich tradition of the Tianjin College of Traditional Chinese Medicine and the scholars who have dedicated themselves to sharing their knowledge with the world. This book will serve that purpose very well.

It is especially important to have this book translated into English since the use of acupuncture and moxibustion in the United States has escalated dramatically over the past few years. It has been acknowledged by excellent western medical schools, as well as the prestigious National Institutes of Health. Contributions to the literature of the discipline advance knowledge and scholars worldwide now have the opportunity to read another excellent reference.

The reader will find the sections on acupuncture and moxibustion techniques, manipulation of the filiform needle and other instruments, as well as micro-acupuncture therapy to be detailed and well documented. Complementing these sections is an extensive appendix with detailed information on point location and manipulation for specific indications. This section provides a quick and useful guide for the practitioner.

I have modified the grammar as little as possible in order to retain the rich and unique style provided by the Chinese translators. It is my firm hope that my efforts have not distorted the rich heritage provided within this book. It is with my utmost respect for the Chinese culture and the profession of Traditional Chinese Medicine that I invite you to benefit from the knowledge presented in this book.

Donald P. Lauda, Ph. D.
Dean, College of Health and Human Services
California State University, Long Beach
Long Beach, California, USA

CONTENTS

Chapter One   Introduction to Acupuncture Therapy ···················· 1

Ⅰ. **Commonly Used Needle Instruments** ································· 1

1. Filiform Needles ··································· 3

   1) The Structure of Filiform Needles

   2) The Gauge of Filiform Needles

   3) The Choice of Filiform Needles

   4) The Check of Filiform Needles

2. Other Needle Apparatuses ························· 4

   Appendix: The Nine Kinds of Needles in Ancient China

   1) Arrowhead-Like Needle

   2) Ovoid-Tip Needle

   3) Blunt Needle

   4) Ensiform Needle

   5) Sword-Like Needle

   6) Round-Shape Needle

   7) Filiform Needle

   8) Long Needle

   9) Large Needle

Ⅱ. **Preparation Before Acupuncture** ························· 7

1. Position of the Patient ··························· 7

   1) Lying Position

   2) Sitting Position

2. Acupoint Location and Its Sterilization ··············· 10

   1) Acupoint Location

   2) Common Sterilization

Ⅲ. **Angle, Direction and Depth of Needle Insertion** ············ 10

1. Angle of Needle Insertion ························· 11

   1) Perpendicular Puncture

   2) Oblique Puncture

3) Horizontal Puncture

2. Direction of Needle Insertion ·· 12

3. Depth of Needle Insertion ··· 12

  1) Varying with the Individuals

  2) Varying with the Acupoint

  3) Varying with the Meridian

  4) Varying with the Disease

  5) Varying with the Season

4. Acupuncture Therapy as in the *Yellow Emperor's Internal Classic* ·············· 14

  1) Nine Types of Needlings

  2) Twelve Methods of Needlings

  3) Five Kinds of Punctures

Ⅳ. **Common Procedure of Acupuncture Therapy** ······················· 22

Ⅴ. **Prevention and Management of Possible Accidents in**

   Acupuncture Therapy ·· 23

1. Acupuncture Syncope ··· 23

2. Sticking of the Needle ·· 23

3. Bending of the Needle ·· 24

4. Breaking of the Needle ··· 25

5. Hematoma ·· 25

6. Infection ··· 26

7. Residual Sensation ··· 26

8. Pricking Injury of Zang-Organs (Viscera) ································· 26

  1) Traumatic Pneumothorax

  2) Piercing Injury of the Heart, Liver, Spleen, Kidney and Other Internal Organs

  3) Piercing Injury of Brain and Spinal Cord

  4) Piercing Injury of the Nerve Trunck

Ⅵ. **Precautions in Acupuncture Therapy** ······························· 28

Ⅶ. **Practicing Methods of Needling Skills** ···························· 29

1. Practice of the Finger Force ··· 29

2. Practice of the Common Manipulations ···································· 30

  1) Practicing Quick Puncturing

  2) Practicing Twirling-Rotating Puncturing

  3) Practicing Lifting-Thrusting Puncturing

  4) Practicing Repeated Lifting-Thrusting Puncturing

3. Self-Needling Test ·· 31

  Appendix: Supplementary Practicing Methods of Needling Skills ·········· 31

  1) Other Practicing Methods of the Finger Force

  2) Palm-Moving and Qi-Training Methods

3) Sitting-Training Method

Ⅷ. **Contraindications in Acupuncture Therapy** ·············· 37

1. Contraindicated Regions ·············· 37

2. Contraindicated Acupoints ·············· 39

3. Contraindication According to the Patient's Condition ·············· 39

4. Provisional Contraindications ·············· 40

Chapter Two   **Manipulations of Filiform Needle in Acupuncture Therapy** ·············· 41

Ⅰ. **Methods of Controlling the Vitality** ·············· 41

Ⅱ. **Methods of Holding the Needle** ·············· 42

1. Holding the Needle with Two Fingers ·············· 43

2. Holding the Needle with Three Fingers ·············· 43

3. Holding the Needle Shaft with Fingers ·············· 43

4. Holding the Needle with Both Hands ·············· 43

Ⅲ. **Methods of Inserting the Needle** ·············· 44

1. Insertion of the Needle with Single Hand ·············· 44

2. Insertion of the Needle with Both Hands ·············· 45

   1) Inserting the Needle with Aid of the Finger of the Pressing Hand

   2) Gripping and Inserting the Needle

   3) Inserting the Needle by Pinching up the Skin

   4) Inserting the Needle by Stretching the Skin

Ⅳ. **Methods of Manipulating the Needle** ·············· 46

1. Lifting and Thrusting Manipulation ·············· 46

2. Twirling and Rotating Manipulation ·············· 47

Ⅴ. **Manipulations of Attaining, Awaiting and Inducing Needling Sensation** ······ 47

1. Attaining of the Needling Sensation ·············· 47

2. Awaiting of the Needling Sensation ·············· 48

3. Inducing of the Needling Sensation ·············· 48

   1) Meridian-Massaging Method

   2) Needle-Flicking Method

   3) Needle-Scraping Method

   4) Needle-Shaking Method

   5) Wing-Spreading Method

   6) Needle-Vibrating Method

   7) Needle-Deepening Method

   8) Needle-Swinging Method

   9) Needle-Thrusting-Drawing Method

Ⅵ. **Manipulations of Directing the Transmission of Needling Sensation** ·············· 51

1. Needle-Tip-Pointing Method ·································· 52

2. Pressing Method ·· 52

3. Needle-Down Method ······································ 52

4. Needle-Bending Method ·································· 53

5. Needle-Tapping Method ·································· 53

6. Needle-Twisting Method ·································· 53

7. Acupoint-Supplementing Method ························ 54

8. Needle-Circling Method ·································· 54

Ⅶ. **Reinforcing and Reducing Manipulations** ·············· 54

1. Reinforcing and Reducing by Lifting and Thrusting the Needle ·········· 55

2. Reinforcing and Reducing by Twirling and Rotating the Needle ·········· 56

3. Reinforcing and Reducing by Rapid and Slow Insertion and Withdrawal of the Needle

··· 57

4. Reinforcing and Reducing by Puncturing along and against the Direction of the Meridian

··· 59

5. Reinforcing and Reducing by Manipulating the Needle in Cooperation with the Patient's Respiration ·· 60

6. Reinforcing and Reducing by Keeping the Needling Hole Open or Close ·········· 60

7. Heat-Inducing Needling(Reinforcing Needling) ·········· 61

8. Cool-Inducing Needling(Reducing Needling) ·········· 62

9. Yin Occluding in Yang(The Reinforcing Containing the Reducing) ·········· 66

10. Yang Occluding in Yin(The Reducing Containing the Reinforcing) ·········· 68

11. Dragon-Tiger Fighting ·································· 68

12. Midnight-Noon Lifting and Thrusting of the Needle ·········· 69

 Appendix 1 Uniform Reinforcing and Reducing Method and Qi-Inducing Method

··· 70

 Appendix 2 The Strong and Weak Stimulation ·········· 71

 Appendix 3 The Other Reinforcing and Reducing Methods ·········· 71

Ⅷ. **Manipulations of Retaining and Withdrawing the Needle** ·········· 71

1. Retaining the Needle ···································· 71

2. Withdrawing the Needle ·································· 72

Ⅸ. **Acupoint-Penetrating Manipulation** ·················· 73

Chapter Three Other Needle Instruments and Their Manipulations in Acupuncture Therapy ·········· 78

Ⅰ. **Acupuncture with the Three-Edged Needle** ·········· 78

1. The Needle Apparatuses ·································· 79

2. Manipulation and Procedure ···························· 79

3. Indications ·· 81

4. Precautions ·· 82

Ⅱ. Acupuncture with the Cutaneous Needle ······························· 82

1. Needle Apparatuses and Preparation before Operation ··················· 83

2. Manipulation and Procedure ·· 83

3. Location of the Tapping ·· 84

　1) Tapping along the Meridian Course

　2) Tapping the Corresponding Acupoints

　3) Tapping the Affected Area

4. Indications ·· 85

5. Precautions ·· 86

Ⅲ. Acupuncture with the Intradermal Needle ··························· 87

1. Needle Apparatuses ·· 87

2. Manipulation and Procedure ·· 87

　1)Manipulation with the Granular(Wheat-Granule-Shaped) Interdermal Needle

　2)Manipulation with the Thumb-Tack(Thumb-Pin-Shaped) Interdermal Needle

3. Indications ·· 88

4. Precautions ·· 88

Ⅳ. Acupuncture with the Electric Needle Apparatuses ··············· 88

1. The Selection of the Needle Instruments, Electric Current and Wave Forms ············· 88

　1) The Types of Electric Stimulators

　2) The Property and Selection of Electric Current

　3) The Selection of the Undulate Wave Forms of the Pulse Electro-Stimulator and Their

　　Functions

2. Manipulation and Procedure ·· 90

　1) Selection and Prescription of the Acupoints

　2) Operation of the Electric Stimulation

3. Indications ·· 91

4. Precautions ·· 91

Ⅴ. Acupuncture with the Cauterized Needle ···························· 92

1. The Needle Apparatuses ·· 92

2. Manipulation and Procedure ·· 92

　1) Selection and Sterilization of Needling Area

　2) Burning of the Needle

　3) Puncturing and Its Depth

3. Indications ·· 93

4. Precautions ·· 93

Ⅵ. Pricking, Cutting, Point-Threading, Point-Catgut-Embedding and Point-Ligation Therapies ·· 94

1. The Pricking Therapy ·· 94

2. The Cutting Therapy 95

3. The Point-Threading, Point-Catgut-Embedding and Point-Ligation Therapies 95

   1) The Point-Threading Therapy

   2) The Point-Catgut-Embedding Therapy

   3) The Point-Ligation Therapy

4. The Acupoint Strong Stimulation Therapy 97

5. Precautions 97

Ⅶ. **Hydro-Acupuncture(Point-Injection) Therapy** 97

1. Manipulations and Procedure 97

2. Indications 98

3. Precautions 98

Appendix   Air Acupuncture(Point-Injection) Therapy 98

Chapter Four   General Introduction to Moxibustion Therapy 99

Ⅰ. **Moxibustion Classification and Its Commonly Used Materials** 99

1. Moxibustion Classification 99

2. Commonly Used Materials for Moxibustion 100

Ⅱ. **Functions of Moxibustion** 101

1. Warming and Dispersing the Cold Evil 101

2. Warming and Dredging the Meridians and Promoting Blood Circulation to Remove Blood Stasis 101

3. Recuparating the Depleted Yang and Rescuing Collapsed Patients 102

4. Relieving Stagnation and Dispersing Accumulated Evils 102

5. Preventing Diseases and Promoting Health 102

Ⅲ. **Precautions for Moxibustion** 102

1. Body Position for Moxibustion 102

2. General Procedure of Moxibustion 102

3. Quantity of Moxibustion 102

4. Management of the Moxibustion Scar 103

5. Contraindication for Moxibustion 103

Chapter Five   Special Introduction to Moxibustion Therapy 104

Ⅰ. **Moxibustion with Moxa Cone** 104

1. Direct Moxibustion 105

   1) Pustula-Forming Moxibustion

   2) Non-Pustula-Forming Moxibustion

2. Indirect Moxibustion 106

   1) Ginger-Partition Moxibustion

   2) Garlic-Partition Moxibustion

    3) Salt-Partition Moxibustion

    4) Herbal-Cake-Partition Moxibustion

Ⅱ. **Moxibustion with Moxa Stick** ·· 108

1. Mild-Warming Moxibustion ·· 108

2. Sparrow-Pecking and Rounding Moxibustions ······················· 108

Ⅲ. **Moxibustion with Moxa on Needle** ································ 110

1. Apparatuses ·· 110

    1) Filiform Needle

    2) Moxa Section

    3) Temperature-Controlling Partition

    4) Heated-Needle Fork

2. Manipulations and Procedure ··· 111

    1) Direct Heated Needle Moxibustion

    2) Indirect Heated Needle Moxibustion

    3) Indications

    4) Precautions

Ⅳ. **Moxibustion with Instruments** ································ 112

1. Apparatus ·· 112

2. Manipulation and Procedure ·· 112

Ⅴ. **Other Types of Moxibustions** ································ 112

1. Taiyi Moxa-Cigar and Thunder-Fire Miraculous Moxibustion ··········· 112

    1) Taiyi Moxa-Cigar Moxibustion

    2) Thunder-Fire Miraculous Moxibustion

2. Crude Herb Moxibustion ·· 113

3. Burning Rush Moxibustion ·· 114

Appendix 1   Moxibustions with Other Materials and Their Functions and Indications

    ·· 115

Appendix 2   Cupping ·· 117

    1) The Classification of Cups

    2) Cupping Manipulation

    3) Applications of Various Cuppings

    4) Indications and Precautions of Cupping

Chapter Six   **Micro-Acupuncture Therapy (Local Acupuncture**
    Therapy) ·· 123

Ⅰ. **Auricular Acupuncture** ·· 123

1. The Auricule and Auricular Points ································ 124

    1) The Relationship of the Ear with the Zang-Fu Organs and Meridian-Collateral System

    2) Anatomical Structure of the Auricule

3) Distribution of the Auricular Points

4) Location and Indications of Commonly Used Ear Points

5) Diagnostic Methods of Auricular Points

2. Clinical Applications of Auricular Acupuncture ·· 136

1) Clinical Indications of Auricular Acupuncture

2) Principles for Selecting Auricular Points

3) Manipulations and Procedure

Ⅱ. **Scalp Acupuncture** ·· 139

1. The Relationship of the Head with the Zang-Fu Organs and

Meridian-Collateral System ··· 139

2. Location and Indications of Stimulation Areas on the Scalp ······················· 140

3. Location and Indications of the Standard Nomenclature of Scalp Acupuncture Lines ··· 143

4. Manipulations and Procedure ·· 146

5. Precautions ··· 147

Ⅲ. **Facial and Nosal Acupuncture** ··· 148

1. The Theoretic Basis of the Facial and Nosal Acupuncture and Their

Point Distribution Areas ·· 148

2. Location and Indications of the Acupoints of Facial Acupuncture ··············· 148

3. Location and Indications of the Acupoints of Nosal Acupuncture ··············· 148

4. Manipulations of the Facial and Nosal Acupuncture ································· 155

5. Precautions ··· 155

Ⅳ. **Occular Acupuncture** ·· 155

1. Occular Distribution Areas ··· 155

2. Manipulation and Procedure ··· 156

3. Acupoints Selection ··· 156

Ⅴ. **Wrist and Ankle Acupuncture** ·· 157

Ⅵ. **Hand and Foot Acupuncture** ··· 159

Ⅶ. **Acupuncture on the Radial Aspect of the Second Metacarpal Bone** ·········· 176

1. Location and Indications of the Acupoints of Radio

Aspect of the Second Metacarpal Bone ·· 176

2. Manipulations of the Acupuncture of the Radio Aspect of the Second Metacarpal Bone

··· 177

Chapter One

Introduction to Acupuncture Therapy

In Traditional Chinese Medicine, acupuncture therapy may be divided into two parts, the general and the specific. The general refers to the practical manipulation of needles after acupoints (or parts) of the body have been selected in light of the differentiation of sign and symptoms, which is also called needling manipulation. The specific refers to the concrete techniques used when acupuncture is administered, where the needling sensation is controlled to attain the desired reinforcing or reducing purpose. This is also named "needling manoeuvre". The ones designed to increase the reinforcing and reducing effects(also called reinforcing and reducing manoeuvre) are the most important.

Acupuncture therapy in the general sense can be studied as follows. (See Fig. 1—1)

I. Commonly Used Needle Instruments

Needles are appliances used to treat diseases. In ancient times, they were usually cuneiform stones called flint needles. In the period of the Warring States(BC 475—221)they were developed into nine types of needles whose length, shape, size, names and usage varied. Present day needles have evolved from the ancient nine needles. They are made of different materials such as gold, silver and stainless steel and their manufacturing technology also varies.

The general sense of Acupuncture Therapy

- Acupuncture with filiform needles
  - Needle appliances
  - Preparation before acupuncture
  - Angle, direction and depth of acupuncture
  - Procedures of acupuncture
    - Needle insertion (needle-holding hand and skin-pressing hand)
    - Needling sensation (spiritual concentration of acupuncturist and full attention of patient)
    - Waiting for and inducing needling sensation
    - Directing needling sensation
    - Reinforcing and reducing manipulations
    - Retaining the needle
    - Withdrawing the needle
  - Prevention and management of abnormal cases in acupuncture
  - Points of attention in acupuncture
  - Practice of acupuncture manipulations
- Acupuncture with other needles
  - Puncture with three-edged needle
  - Puncture with cutaneous needle
  - Puncture with warmed needle
  - Puncture with cauterized needle
  - Puncture with thick needle
  - Hydro-needling
  - Puncture with awn needle
  - Needle-pricking
  - Puncture with blunt needle
  - Puncture with pottery needle
  - Laquer needling
  - Puncture with electrical needle
  - Obstructed needling
  - Collateral-pricking (blood-letting puncture)
  - Puncture with laser needle
  - Acupuncture anesthesia

Fig. 1—1   The Content of Acupuncture Therapy

1. Filiform Needles

The Filiform needle is one of the nine type of needles used in ancient times. Since its shape and structure is ideal to puncture the points on any part of the body, the filiform needle is the most commonly used in clinical practice. Acupuncture therapy in past dynasties primarily utilized this kind of needle.

1) The Structure of Filiform Needles

The filiform needle used today is usually made of stainless steel. Its structure may be divided into five parts which are as follows: (See Fig. 1—2)

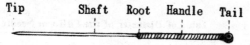

Tip   Shaft   Root   Handle   Tail

Fig. 1—2   The Structure of Filiform Needle

A. The needle tip——Refers to the sharp front part of the needle, also named Zhenmang (needle awn)

B. The needle body——Refers to the main part of the needle between the tip and root, also called Zhenti(needle shaft)

C. The needle root——Refers to the conjunction of the body and handle.

D. The needle handle——Refers to the part behind the root of the needle, which is the area where the needle is held and force is exerted. Usually it is wound with metal wire so as to hold the needle easily.

E. The needle tail——Refers to the end of the needle handle. It is also the part where mugwort floss is applied when warm needling with moxibustion is administered.

2) The Gauge of Filiform Needles

The gauge of the filiform needle is determined on the basis of the length and diameter of the needle body. In the clinic, the choice of different gauges should be made according to the treatment given.

Generally all the filiform needles listed above should be utilized in the clinic, with the 25—27mm long(1—3 cun) and size 28# —30# (0.32mm—0.38mm in calibre) used most widely.

3) The Choice of the Filiform Needles

(1) The tip should not be unduly sharp. It should be round but not blunt. The one shaped like a pine needle is regarded as the best. Attention should be paid to any improper minute hooks or divided tips.

(2) The body must be erect, smooth, taut, elastic and flexible. If there are traces or specks of rust on the needle, or the needle is crooked and twisted, it should no longer be used.

(3) The root must be firm and fixed. It should not be loose or rusted.

(4) The handle should be closely and evenly wound with a metallic thread. It is not advisable to wind it excessively long or short.

Tab. 1—1   **Table of Length of the Filiform Needle**

Old gauge (cun) New gauge (mm)		0.5	1	1.5	2	2.5	3	4	4.5	5	6
Length of the body		15	25	40	50	65	75	100	115	125	150
Length of the handle	Long	25	35	40	40	40	40	55	55	55	56
	Medium		30	35	35						
	Short	20	25	25	30	30	30	40	40	40	40

Tab. 1—2   **Table of Diameter of the Filiform Needle**

Size	26	27	28	29	30	31	32	33	34	35
Diameter(mm)	0.45	0.42	0.38	0.34	0.32	0.30	0.28	0.26	0.23	0.22

4) The Check of the Filiform Needles

(1) Make sure the tip has no curly ends or minute hooks. The check can be conducted by twirling the needle handle with the thumb and index finger. Simultaneously with the third finger touching the needle tip frequently. Generally, if the tip is crooked, the problem can be detected immediately by the third finger. For sterilized filiform needles, the detection of minute hooks in the tip can be made by holding a cotton ball in the left hand with the right hand holding the handle of the needle with the tip of it in the alcohol cotton ball. If some cotton fibre attaches to the tip when the needle is withdrawn from the ball, it shows that the tip has the minute hook.

(2) Make sure whether the needle body has any specks of dust, rust, bends or is broken. To check the needle, use one hand to hold the handle of the needle and the thumb and second finger of the other hand to slightly rub the needle body up and down. If you do not have a smooth sensation while doing so, it indicates that there are some places where there is rust or bends.

(3) Make sure the handle of the needle is not loose. With one hand holding the handle and the other hand the body, apply force or turn it forwards and backwards. If the handle is loose, it is easily noticed.

2. Other Needle Apparatuses

At present, apart from the filiform needles, the other commonly used needles in the clinic are the three-edged needle, cutaneous needle, intradermal needle, cauterized needle and hydro-needle. More details about them will be presented in following chapters.

Appendix: The Nine Kinds of Needles in Ancient China

The nine kinds of needles originated in ancient China and they were mentioned in many chapters in the *Internal Classic*(内经, Nei Jing). Reference is made to nine kinds of needles of different shapes suitable for the treatment of various diseases. In many chapters of the *Internal Classic*(内经, Nei Jing) there are records about the nine needles. For instance, the *Miraculous Pivot* (灵枢, Ling Shu) says that, "The nine needles differ in shape and length but they have their own advantages and objects". Unfortunately, until now, no material samples have been found.

Du Sijing(杜思敬）, a physician in the Yuan Dynasty was the first to draw pictures of the ancient nine needles. Later, in the Ming and Qing dynasties, there were many records which gave descriptions of the ancient nine needles, though the pictures of the nine needles were all different in shape and size. In 1986, restored models of the ancient nine needles were developed in Suzhou which were appraised and authenticated by both experts and archaeologists. (See Fig. 1—3)

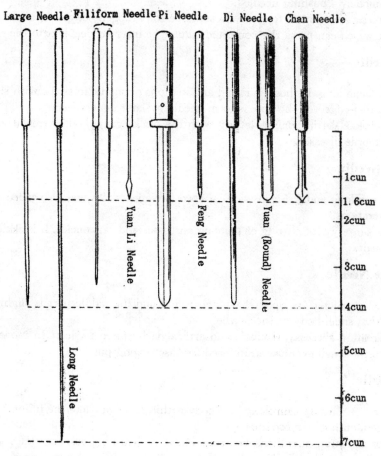

Fig. 1—3   The Nine Kinds of Needles in Ancient China

1) Arrowhead-Like Needle

A. Shape: 1.6 cun long, like an arrowhead. Its head is large but its tip is sharp. It becomes small 1/3 centimeter from the end of the needle, forming the tip. The cutaneous needle is the evolution of this needle.

B. Usage: For superficial pricking and treatment of febrile diseases, using the blood-letting method.

2) Ovoid-Tip Needle

A. Shape: 1.6 cun long. Its body is cylindrical and its tip is oval. It was later developed into the round-tip needle.

B. Usage: For massaging the body surface or the acupuncture points and to treat diseases due to pathogens lingering in muscles without impairing the muscles. It is a kind of massaging and rubbing instrument.

3) Blunt Needle

A. Shape: 3. 5 cun long. Its tip, like a millet, is round, short and slightly sharp. It has been improved into the modern "pushing needle".

B. Usage: Pressing meridians to treat diseases due to pathogens lingering in the meridians. It is an instrument which can press the point and cannot be inserted deeply into the muscles.

4) Ensiform Needle

A. Shape: 1. 6 cun long. Its body is round and its tip is prismatic in shape with sharp edges. It was also called three-edged or the tri-ensiform needle by later generations.

B. Usage: For blood-letting or pus-letting with the pricking method to treat abscesses, carbuncles and acute febrile diseases.

5) Sword-Like Needle

A. Shape: 4 cun long and 2. 5 cun wide, shaped like a sword. It was also called sword-head needle in later generations.

B. Usage: In surgery, for cutting or piercing abscesses and carbuncles. It is a kind of surgical cutting instrument.

6) Round-Shape Needle

A. Shape: 1. 6 cun long. Its tip is sharp and round and its middle part is slightly larger in contrast with the thin small body of the needle.

B. Usage: Treating abscess, carbuncle and arthralgia by piercing deep. In modern times, it has been made into the small eyebrow knife used for discharging pus.

7) Filiform Needle

A. Shape: From 1. 6 to 3. 6 cun long. Its body is thin and fine, like the filiform, and its tip is tenuous, like the mouth of a mosquito.

B. Usage: For activating meridians and collaterals, replenishing essence and supplementing qi, treating febrile disease and arthralgia. It is the most commonly used needle in clinics today.

8) Long Needle

A. Shape: 7 cun long. Its body is comparatively long with a sharp tip. It is an elongated or filiform needle.

B. Usage: Treating various syndromes of "pathogens in the deep interior with distal arthralgia" such as chronic rheumatism and sciatica by deep needling. It was called "Huantiao Needling (环跳针)" by later generations which means that the needle was inserted at the Huantiao(GB 30) point. Later, it was improved to the awn needle.

9) Large Needle

A. Shape: 4 cun long. Its body is relatively thick with a blunt tip. It is the long form of an ensiform needle.

B. Usage: For removing water retention, treating anasarca. Later generations use it as a cauterized needle to treat scrofula and mammary abscesses.

The classification of the ancient nine needles and their applications are summarized as follows. (See Tab. 1—3)

Tab. 1－3 **Table of Classification of the Ancient Nine Needles in Application**

Name of needle	Use	Clinical application
1. Arrow-head needle	Superficial pricking	Febrile disease which occurs in the surface
2. Ovoid tip needle	Massaging the body surface of the muscular layers with it (a kind of massaging appliance)	Muscular diseases
3. Blunt needle	Pressing the exterior of the meridians or blood vessels. (pressing the meridian or blood vessels moderately just to drive the pathogen away)	Vascular disease marked by asthenia and deficiency of qi, febrile disease and headache
4. Ensiform needle	Pricking the point or superficial vein for blood-letting (i. e. the three-edged needle)	Abscess, carbuncle, intractable illness and muscular disease
5. Sword-like needle	Cutting or piercing the abscess or carbuncle to discharge pus (a kind of surgical appliance)	Abscess or carbuncle with purulence
6. Round-shaped needle	A sharp and thick needle, used for quick pricking	Abscess, carbuncle, arthralgia (Bi-)syndrome
7. Filiform needle	The most widely used needle in treating febrile diseases, abscess, carbuncle and arthralgia	Strengthening the body's resistance and eliminating pathogenic factors; miscellaneous diseases of internal medicine
8. Long needle	Used in the muscular parts of the body	The intractable arthralgia in the deep part of the body
9. Large needle	Used to needle the areas near the big joints of four extremities	Treating arthralgia

Ⅱ. **Preparation Before Acupuncture**

1. **Position of the Patient**

In clinical acupuncture treatment, proper position of the patient directly influences the correct location of the acupoint and the curative effect of acupuncture. When puncturing, the patient should take a position in which the acupuncturist can easily manipulate the needles and the patient feels comfortable and natural and can maintain the position for a relatively long time. In the clinic, there are two common positions, lying and sitting. Generally, the lying position is used for patients who are old, weak and nervous about the needling therapy. The lying position may prevent the occurrence of acupuncture syncope and other accidents. Now the commonly used positions are respectively related as follows:

1) Lying Position

(1) Supine position: Suitable for puncturing the points on the forehead, face, neck, chest, abdomen, upper limbs, anterior surface and lateral sides of lower limbs, hands and feet. (See Fig. 1—4)

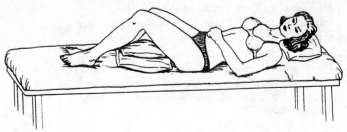

Fig. 1—4   The Supine Posture

(2) Lateral recumbent position: Suitable for puncturing the points on the lateral sides of the hands, chest, abdomen, buttock and lower extremities. (See Fig. 1—5)

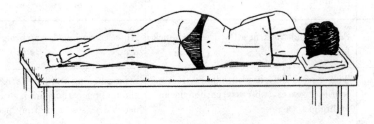

Fig. 1—5   The Lateral Recumbent Posture

(3) Prone position: Suitable for puncturing the points on the nape, shoulder, back, lumbosacral and posterior and lateral portions of lower extremities. (See Fig. 1—6)

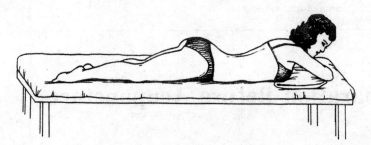

Fig. 1—6   The Prone Posture

2) Sitting Position

(1) Supine sitting position: Fit for the points on forehead, face, neck and upper part of the chest. (See Fig. 1—7)

(2) Prone sitting position: Fit for the points on vertex, occiput, posterior nape, shoulder and back. (See Fig. 1—8)

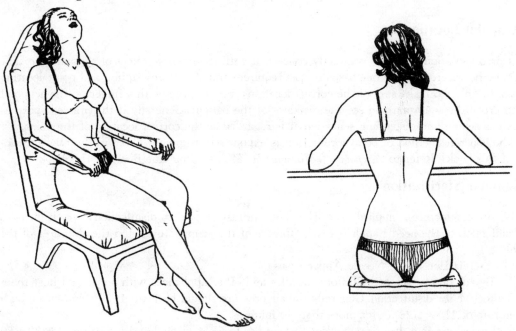

Fig. 1—7　The Supine Sitting Posture　　　　　**Fig. 1—8　The Prone Sitting Posture**

On the lying or sitting position, the four limbs should be in an appropriate flexion posture. For instance, if the points on the palmar surface of the upper limbs are selected, supine palmar posture should be taken; if the points on the dorsal part of the upper limbs are to be punctured, a prone palmar posture should be taken. If the points on the lateral sides of the lower limbs and the areas of knee joints are to be punctured, the genuflexion posture should be often taken. In addition, there are other points which require specific postures. For example, the *Miraculous Pivot* (灵枢, Ling Shu) says, "If the point Dubi(ST 35) is punctured, flexion posture should be taken instead of stretching posture, and if the points Shangguan(GB 3) and Xiaguan(ST 7) are punctured, stretching posture should be taken. " "For the point Zhongfeng(LR 4)··· the foot should be shaken and rocked when selected and punctured. " "For the point Quchi(LI 11)···the arm should be flexed. " The *Miraculous Pivot*(灵枢, Ling Shu)says, "If the point of Zusanli(ST 36) is chosen, a foot-lower posture should be taken; If Shangjuxu(ST 37) point is chosen, a foot-raised posture should be used; If Weiyang(BL 39)point is chosen, both flexion and stretching postures should be taken; If Weizhong(BL 40) point is chosen, flexion posture is taken; If Yanglingquan (GB 34) point is chosen, a squatting posture is taken with the upper part of the body being erect and both knees being at the same level and select the point at the lateral side of Weiyang(BL 39). " And the *A-B Classic of Acupuncture and Moxibustion*(甲乙经, Jia Yi Jing)says, "For Huantiao(GB 30)point··· the latericumbent position is taken with the lower leg stretched and upper leg flexed. "*Mingtang Moxibustion*(明堂灸经, Ming Tang Jiu Jing) also says, "For Yifeng (ST 17)···the patient should open the mouth by biting an ancient Chinese copper coin when this point is selected. " Zhen Quan(甄权, Zhen Quan)says, "For Shaohai(HT 3)···the hand should be flexed towards the head. " The information presented above all indicates that different distribution of the points on the body determines the variable positions or postures in point selection.

2. Acupoint Location and Its Sterilization

1) Acupoint Location

Correct location of points is directly concerned with the curative effect of acupuncture. The point may be selected one by one based on the requirements of the prescription and point-locating method. In order to make sure of the correct location, one can press with a finger on the acupoint area to probe the sensation and see the response of the patient. Generally if the pressed spot has an obvious aching and distending sensation, it is regarded as the correct location of the point.

The concrete method of point localization is expounded in greater detail in the relevant sections of this book. Refer to *Acupoints & Moxibustion*(经穴篇, Jing Xue Pian) of this book.

2) Common Sterilization

When acupuncture is applied, special attention must be paid to disinfection, which includes the disinfection of the needle appliances, the fingers of the acupuncturist and the skin area of the patient.

(1) Sterilization of the Needle Apparatuses

A. By autoclave: Wrap the filiform needles and other appliances with gauze and heat them in the autoclave for disinfection. Generally the air pressure should be 1.0—1.5kg/cm with a high temperature of 115— 123 ℃ for more than 30 minutes.

B. By soaking in a disinfectant: Put the needles in 75% alcohol and soak them for 30—60 minutes; then take out and dry them for use. They may also be put into a disinfectant solution prepared with 1% bromogeramine and 0.5% sodium nitrite for 1—2 hours.

In addition, the trays and tweezers which are directly in contact with the filiform needle should also be sterilized. The disinfected needles must be placed in a sterile tray with a lid or covered with antiseptic gauze.

(2) Sterilization of the clinician's Fingers

The hands, esp. the fingers of the acupuncturist should be first washed clean with soap, or rubbed with alcohol cotton-balls before needling is administered.

(3) Sterilization of the Needling Area

Swab the skin area which is to be punctured in a round and outward fashion with 75% alcohol cotton-balls from the needling point to its surrounding area or swab the area first with 2% iodine tincture, and then, after it has dried slightly, remove the iodine by circling the area outwards with 75% alcohol cotton ball. After sterilization, the needling area must be kept clean and prevented from being contaminated again. At present, disposable filiform needles, which are being popularized, are advantageous in preventing cross infection. They should be considered for use though their cost is comparatively higher.

III. Angle, Direction and Depth of Needle Insertion

In the process of the administration of acupuncture, mastery over the angle, direction and depth of needling is the key link in obtaining the needling sensation, increasing the therapeutic effect and preventing the occurrence of accidents. Accuracy in acupoint selection not only refers to the correct location of acupoint on the skin, but also means the proper angle, direction and depth of the needling. Only when they are appropriately combined with each other, can the therapeutic effect be fully achieved. The reason is that when the same point is punctured, if the angle, direction or depth of needling change, the needle may reach different tissue and different needling sensation can occur, thus, bringing about a different therapeutic effect. Take point Jianjing(GB 21) for example, if it is punctured at different angles, needling response may occur at different sites, as a result, different diseases can be treated. If the needle is inserted with the tip facing anteriorly, the needling response radiate to the chest, and mammary diseases can be treated. If the needle is inserted with the tip outwards, making the needling response radiate to the acromion, shoulder disease may be treated. If the needle is inserted with the tip backwards, making the response radiate to the scapular region, pedal flaccidity and pain may be treated. Also, when the point Sanyinjiao(SP 6) is punctured, different needling depth may cause the response to move along the meridians of Foot Shaoyin, Foot Taiyin and Foot Jueyin, thereby treating different diseases. The degree of proficiency is closely related to the command in the angle, direction and depth one uses in acupuncture. In the clinic, the choice of the angle, direction and depth should be made with flexibility according to the condition of the needling area, requirements of treatment and the patients' different constitutions.

1. Angle of Needle Insertion

It refers to the angle formed by the shaft of the needle inserted and the skin surface punctured. The degree of the angle is mainly dependent upon the characteristic of the region where the acupoint lies and the requirements of the treatment. Generally there are three kinds: the perpendicular, the oblique and horizontal puncture. (See Fig. 1—9).

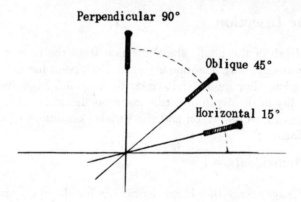

Perpendicular 90°

Oblique 45°

Horizontal 15°

Fig. 1—9   The Angle of the Needle Insertion

1) Perpendicular Puncture

When the needle enters into the skin, it should stand at an angle of 90 degrees to the skin surface and is inserted perpendicularly into the point. This kind of needling is suitable for most points in the body, especially those in a thick muscular region.

2) Oblique Puncture

When the needle enters into the skin, it should stand at an angle of 45 degrees to the skin surface and is inserted obliquely into the point. This kind of needling is applicable to the points which are unfit to be punctured deeply.

3) Horizontal Puncture

When the needle enters into the skin, it should stand at an angle of 15 degrees to the skin surface. It is inserted horizontally under the skin, and is also called transverse needling. This kind is suitable for the acupoint on the parts of the body where the muscles are thin.

2. Direction of Needle Insertion

This refers to area or region of the body towards which the needle tip is directed when the needle is inserted into the skin. It has a close connection with the angle of the insertion. In general, the direction of insertion is determined by the circulating direction of the meridians and the distribution of points and tissues the needle is supposed to reach. Only through good control of the puncturing direction, can the needling effect be enhanced, ensuring the safety of acupuncture. In the clinic, in light of the need to direct the transmission of the needling sensation and with a view to directing "the qi to the diseased area, " the tip of needle should be inserted into the diseased part. Sometimes, in view of the need to reinforce, or reduce, or with the view to "tonifying or reducing by puncturing along or against the direction of the meridian, " the needle tip is required to be inserted along or against the direction of the meridian. In practical applications, in order to ensure the safety of acupuncture, the inserting direction of the needle tip, in accordance to the distribution of the acupoints, has been stipulated. For example, when the point Yamen(DU 15) is punctured, the needle tip should be directed to the mouth and lip of the patient. When some points on the back are punctured, the tip should be pointed towards the spinal column.

3. Depth of Needle Insertion

This refers to the depth of the needle shaft insertion from the time it is inserted into the body until the time when the needling sensation is gained. Each point has its own criterion for the depth of the needle insertion. (For more details, refer to *Acupoints* & *Meridians* (经穴篇)) In clinical application, flexibility in the depth of needle insertion should be taken in accordance with different patients, diseases, acupoints, season and the variable conditions of both circulation and distribution of the meridians.

1) Varying with the Individuals

(1) Varying with the age: Since the old are deficient in blood and qi, and children have premature yin and yang due to their tender viscera, they are not fit to be deeply punctured. For those who are young and strong with sufficient blood and qi, appropriate deep puncture may be conducted. *Miraculous Pivot*(灵枢, Ling Shu) says, "For infants and emaciated people, shallow and quick puncture is done; for strong and fat people, deep and retained puncture is done".

(2) Varying with the constitution: People differ greatly in constitution and physique and they are characterized by corpulence, emaciation, sturdiness and weakness. For the person who is emaciated with a weak body, it is appropriate to administer shallow needling. For the person who is big with a sturdy body, it is suitable to administer deep needling. As *Plain Questions*(素问, Su Wen) says, "When puncturing, it is necessary to consider the patient's physique and constitution so as to regulate the imbalance due to deficiency or excess of qi. "

2) Varying with the Acupoint

In general, for the acupoints on the head, face, chest and back, shallow needling is used. For the acupoints on the four limbs, buttock and abdomen, appropriate deep needling is used. In the clinic, the clinician must follow the principle that if the acupoint is a shallow one, it is punctured superficially, and if it is a deep one, it is punctured deeply. Only by doing so, can the curative effect of needling be exerted along with the guarantee of safety. As *A Collection of Gems in Acupuncture and Moxibustion*(针灸聚英,Zhen Jiu Ju Ying)says, "If asked how deep the needle is inserted into the Liao-points…,the body has both superficial and deep muscles and diseases are located shallow or deep. If the muscles are thick,deep puncture is used and if the muscles are thin,shallow puncture is used."

3) **Varying with the Meridian**

The depth of needling and the property of Yin and Yang of the meridian which is to be punctured should also be considered. In general, Yang meridian pertains to the exterior and shallow needling is appropriate. Yin meridian pertains to the interior and it is fit to be punctured deeply. As *Miraculous Pivot*(灵枢, Ling Shu) says, "If Yin meridian is punctured,the needle is inserted deeply and retained and if Yang meridian is punctured, the needle is inserted shallowly and withdrawn rapidly."

4) **Varying with the Disease**

Generally speaking, shallow puncture is suitable for Yang syndrome, exterior syndrome and new diseases; and deep puncture is used for Yin syndrome,interior syndrome and chronic or protracted diseases. As *Plain Questions*(素问,Su Wen) says, "Disease may be manifested as either floating or deep pulse, and needling falls into shallow or deep punctures." *Miraculous Pivot*(灵枢,Ling Shu) also says, "For a patient with excess pulse,deep needling is used…,for a patient with deficient pulse,shallow needling is used." "Patients with pains,pertaining to Yin, are punctured deeply;patients with itching,pertaining to Yang, are punctured shallow." These all stress the importance of the depth of acupuncture.

5) **Varying with the Season**

Since the physiological and pathological states of the human body are connected closely with the seasons,the depth of acupuncture must vary with the seasons. *Plain Questions*(素问,Su Wen,)points out that, "Puncture differs in spring, summer, autumn and winter." *Classic of Medical Problems*(难经, Nan Jing) says that, "In spring and summer, Yang-qi is high and the human qi is also superficial,so shallow puncture is used. In autumn and winter, Yin-qi is down and the human qi is also deep,so deeper puncture is used." The all show that the depth of needling should correspond with the Yin-Yang of Heaven and Earth and must vary with the changing seasons.

The depth of needling can also be regulated according to the occurrence of different needling sensations. For the patient who is sensitive to the needling,shallow needling is used. For the patient who is not so sensitive to the needling,appropriate deep needling is used,or the direction and angle of needling are changed. Generally speaking,the depth of needling also varies with the different habit and manipulation of the clinician,and the depth of needling of each point conducted by each person is not immutable. So the clinician should master it in accordance with given conditions.

In summary,the angle,direction and depth of acupuncture have a close mutual relationship. Usually, deep needling is conducted with the perpendicular method and shallow needling is done with the oblique or horizontal method. The direction of needling is dependent on the angle of the insertion,and at the same time, the direction of the puncture is one of the important factors in determining the depth of puncture. For the points in the region of the medullary bulb, eyes, chest and back,since they lie in an area where important organs are located, special attention should be paid to the angle,direction and depth when needling so as to avoid the occurrence of medical accidents.

4. Acupuncture Therapy as in the *Yellow Emperor's Internal Classic*（内 经，Nei Jing）

There are nine types of needling, twelve methods of needling and five kinds of puncture mentioned in *Miraculous Pivot*（灵枢，Ling Shu）which were considered in past dynasties to be the representative of the acupuncture therapy in the *Internal Classic*（内经，Nei Jing）. However, not all of them were concerned with the techniques of acupuncture. They mainly dwelt on the acupoint selection, acupoint prescription, the depth of puncture and varied needling techniques. These are described as follows：

1) Nine Types of Needlings

Miraculous Pivot（灵枢，Ling Shu）says, "There are nine types of needling in respond to nine kinds of changes." "Changes" here refer to the pathogenic changes of different nature. The main contents of the nine types of needling discuss the application of different acupoint selection and needling techniques with nine kinds of pathogenic changes.

(1) Shu-Point Needling：Shu-point needling means puncturing the Ying(spring) and Shu (stream) points on the meridians and the visceral Shu points on the back. This is a point-selection method for treating visceral diseases. If one of the visceras is diseased, the Ying(spring) and Shu(stream) points, which are related to its meridians and located below the elbows and knees, as well as the back-shu points, which corresponding to the organ, are selected for puncture. *Plain Questions*（素问，Su Wen）says, "In case that the visceras are diseased, they are treated by dealing with the Shu-points," which also indicates the same meaning as above.

(2) Distant-Needling：Distant-needling means puncturing the points in the lower limbs for disease in the upper part of the body. This is a corresponding meridian point-selection. The six-fu organs lie in the trunk of the body while their He-(sea) points are in the lower limbs. When a disease occurs in the upper part of the body, the He-(sea) points(also called Fu-organ points) in the lower limbs are selected for puncture. In addition, distant-needling also refers to Shu-point needling which means that the pathogenic changes of the six fu-organs can be treated by dealing with the Shu(stream) points which correspond to these organs. All the diseases of the sense organs, of the trunk and viscera can be treated by choosing acupoints below the elbow and knees. For example, for headache, choose Taichong(LR 3) and Zhiyin(BL 67); for toothache, choose Hegu(LI 4)and Neiting(ST 44).

(3) Meridian Needling：Meridian needling means puncturing the affected area along the meridians. That is, puncturing the points on the meridians proximal to the affected area where stagnation and obstruction of qi and blood often occurs(marked by blood stasis, scleroma and tenderness). This is a kind of site-determination method in acupuncture, often used to treat diseases on meridians and collaterals.

(4) Collateral Needling：Collateral needling means puncturing the subcutaneous small blood vessels. This is a needling technique which causes bleeding by pricking the superficial blood vessels. *Plain Questions*（素问，Su Wen）says, "If the disease is concerned with blood, the treatment is to puncture the collateral blood capillary." This needling is, in fact, the method for treating excess syndrome or heat syndrome by pricking the small blood vessels to cause bleeding. In addition to this, blood-letting with three-edged needles and cupping therapies can also be used.

(5) Intermuscular Needling：Intermuscular needling means puncturing the space between two muscles. With this technique, the needle is inserted directly into the muscular area. "Intermuslular" here just refers to the area where the muscles are thick and the muscular layers are visible. All the arthralgia-Bi syndrome and pains caused by pathogenic factors which are stored in muscles, or other old disorders, are treated by inserting the needles deeply into the diseased area in order to regulate its meridian qi and dispel the pathogenic factors.

(6) Drainage Needling: Drainage needling means draining pus with the sword-shaped needle. This is a method to evacuate the pus or blood from an abscess, boil or carbuncle by incision with a sword-shaped needle so as to dissipate pathogenic heat.

(7) Skin Needling: Skin needling means puncturing the numb and painful skin superficially. It is a shallow cutaneous puncturing method, used to treat affected areas where the pathogenic factors lie exteriorly and superficially. The current cutaneous needles, which are widely used, have improved this kind of skin needling and greatly enlarge the scopy of treatment.

(8) Contralateral Needling: Contralateral needling means puncturing the right side of the body for left-sided disease and puncturing the left side for right-sided disease. This is a point-selection method which involves selecting points contralateral to the affected side. All the twelve regular meridians of the human body have their own crossing points of the left and right sides. For instance, the three Yang meridians of the hand and foot all cross and converge at the Dazhui (DU 14) point on Du meridian. The three Yin meridians of the foot also cross and converge at the points Zhongji(RN 3)and Guanyuan(RN 4) on Ren meridian, so their meridian qi can be interchanged bilaterally. Thus, the disorders on the left side of the body can be treated by selecting the points on the right-sided meridian while the disorders on the right side can be treated by selecting the points on the left-sided meridian.

(9) Cauterized Needling: Cauterized needling means puncturing the numb and painful sites with a red-hot needle. This is a method in which a red-hot needle is inserted into the affected part and withdrawn quickly. It is applicable for the diseases such as cold-arthralgia, numbness with pain, scrofula and cellulitis.

As a whole, the contents of the nine types of needling may be summarized as follows. (See Tab. 1－4)

2) Twelve Methods of Needling

It is recorded in *Miraculous Pivot*(灵枢, Ling Shu) that, "In acupuncture there are twelve needling methods which correspond to the twelve meridians of the body". This means that during acupuncture treatment there are twelve rules to be noted which accordingly can treat twelve kinds of diseases.

(1) Paired Needling: Paired needling means pressing with both of the hands the painful area of the chest and the corresponding area on the back of the body and puncturing the two areas obliquely with one needle each, primarily used for treating angina pectoris. This technique is conducted by palpating the chest area, which corresponds to the Front-Mu points, with one hand and the same area on the back, which corresponds to the Back-shu points, with the other hand; then inserting needles at the pressed-painful points on both sides. This kind of front and back, or Yin and Yang, paired technique is also called "even" or "Yin-Yang" needling. In clinical treatment, Back-shu and Front-shu points are often used in combination to cure visceral diseases, which also belongs to paired needling.

(2) Trigger Needling: Trigger needling means puncturing a painful trigger point with a needle and retaining it there until another painful trigger point is found; then withdrawing the first needle and puncturing the second trigger point. By calling it trigger needling, we mean it is a technique used to puncture again after the withdrawal of the needle, which is often used to treat wandering pains and other diseases. In clinic, the needle may first be inserted at the painful area the patient complains of, then, after administering the needling manipulations, inquire about the patient's condition, or press the skin along the course of the wandering pain with left hand. If the pain stops, the needle is withdrawn and inserted again at another painful trigger point.

(3) Lateral Needling(Relaxing Needling): Lateral needling means puncturing perpendicularly near the painful muscle and manipulating the needle up and down, anteriorly and posteriorly, right and left in order to relax the muscle. This is a technique to insert the needle perpendicularly and deeply on one side of the painful muscle, shaking it all around, lifting and thrusting it to

dispel pathogenic qi and promoting the flow of qi in the meridians. It is applicable for diseases of muscles with spasm and pain.

Tab. 1－4   Table of Nine Types of Needlings

Nine types of needling	Principle of point selection	Remarks
Shu-point needling	Puncturing the Ying (spring) and Shu (stream) points on the different meridians as well as the visceral Shu points on the back	Selecting the Ying (spring), Shu (stream) and visceral Shu point on the back. (Acupoint selection method)
Distant-needling	Puncturing the Fu-organ (He (sea) points) in the lower limbs of the body when the disease occurs in the upper part of the body	Selecting the points which are far from the affected part; selecting the points in the lower limbs of the body though the disease exists in the upper part of the body. (Acupoint selection method)
Meridian needling	Puncturing the points on meridians proximal to the affected area where stasis and obstruction of qi and blood occur.	Selecting the points on the corresponding meridians proximal to the affected part. (Acupoint selection method)
Collateral needling	Puncturing the subcutaneous small blood vessels	Selecting the points on the superficial blood vessels and puncturing the points to cause bleeding. (Blood-letting by pricking collaterals)
Intermuscular needling	Puncturing the space between two muscles	Selecting the points between the muscular layers of the affected area. (Depth of acupuncture)
Drainage needling	Evacuating the pus with a sword-shaped needle	Surgical drainage of pus (Surgical discharge of pus)
Skin needling	Puncturing the numb and painful skin superficially	Shallow skin puncture (Depth of puncture)
Opposing needling	Puncturing the points contralateral to the affected side	Crossing selection of points (Acupoint selection method)
Cauterized needling	Puncturing numb and painful areas with a red-hot needle	Selecting the points where the pain or numbness occurs (Fire puncture)

(4) Triple Needling: Triple needling means puncturing the center of the affected part with one needle and its two sides with another two needles, to treat the affection of a relatively small and deep area caused by cold. This is a technique to insert one needle at the center of the affected part and then, another two needles on the both sides (each one for each side) of the needle. Since three needles are needed at the same time in this treatment, this needling is also called "simultaneous-triple needling."(See Fig. 1－10)

(5) Centro-Square Needling: Centro-square needling means puncturing the center of the affected area superficially with one needle and placing another four needles around it in a square shape, and is indicated for cases of relatively widespread and superficial cold arthralgia. With this kind of needling, we insert one needle at the center of the affected part superficially, and then, insert another four needles around it. This comparatively superficial and scattered puncture is called centro-square needling. The present tapping technique around the acupoint with cutaneous

needles has evolved from this kind of needling. (See Fig. 1—11)

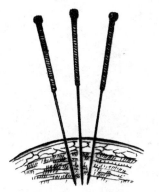

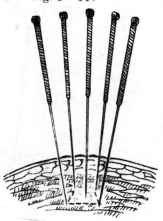

Fig. 1—10 **The Triple Needling**   Fig. 1—11 **The Centro-Square Needling**

(6) Perpendicular Needling: Perpendicular needling means lifting the skin and puncturing subcutaneously but not deeply, for cases of superficial cold arthralgia. This kind of needling does not mean inserting the needle vertically but refers to the skin needling or horizontal needling of modern times. It is often used in the shallow muscular regions and is indicated for the affection of a relative shallow area caused by cold.

(7) Deep Perpendicular Needling: Deep perpendicular needling means thrusting and lifting the needle perpendicularly and deeply with only a few points selected, applicable for cases of excess qi and heat. This is a technique to insert the needle vertically and deeply to wait for the coming of the needling sensation and then, after gaining the sensation, withdraw it perpendicularly and slowly. Only a few points are selected when this technique is used. This kind of needling can dredge the meridians and dispel pathogenic qi.

(8) Short-Thrusting Needling: Short-thrusting needling means inserting the needle directly to the bone with a slight shaking, then lifting and thrusting it to scrape the bone, indicated for osseous rheumatism. With this technique, we thrust the needle slowly, slightly shaking its body to reach the bone, where the needle is lifted and thrusted to scrape the bone. This is often used to treat rheumatism involving the bone.

(9) Superficial Needling: Superficial needling means puncturing superficially lateral to the affected part to treat muscular spasm due to cold. This technique administers a shallow puncture on the sides of the affected part. This is mainly used for treating muscular spasm due to attack of pathogenic cold. The present embedding-needle therapy has evolved from this kind of needling. Superficial, skin and centro-square needlings fall into the category of shallow needling, but skin needling lays emphasis on shallow puncture with less needles. Centro-square needling lays stress on shallow puncture with more needles while the superficial needling lays stress on shallow puncture with the needle inserted obliquely.

(10) Yin Needling: Yin needling means puncturing bilaterally Taixi(KI 3) of the kidney meridian of Foot-Shaoyin behind the medial malleolus of the foot for cases of cold syncope. This is a technique to puncture points on both lateral sides simultaneously. It is used for treating the syncope caused by cold. If the disease occurs in the Shaoyin meridian and manifests as cold limbs, sunken and weak pulse and other cold symptoms, they can be treated by puncturing bilaterally point Taixi(KI 3) of the Kidney meridian of foot-Shaoyin.

(11) Proximal Needling: Proximal needling means inserting the needles in pairs, one in the meridian point and the other in the collateral point, for treating chronic rheumatic diseases due to pathogenic dampness. This is a technique to puncture the affected part vertically and laterally

with one needle each. It is applicable to treat stubborn arthralgia which is characterized by obvious tenderness and immobility. (See Fig. 1—12)

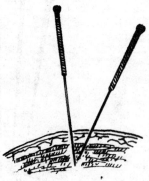

Fig. 1—12   **The Proximal**
Needling

(12) Repeated Shallow Needling: Repeated shallow needling means puncturing the affected part superficially and repeatedly with more than one needle to cause bleeding. This technique requires several needles to be inserted and withdrawn vertically and superficially to cause bleeding of the affected part, and is used for treating carbuncles and erysipelas. It belongs to the category of blood-letting due to shallow puncture. This kind of needling is similar to the collateral needling of the nine types of needling and the leopard-spot puncture of the five sorts of needling in ancient China.

The contents of the twelve types of needling may be summarized as follows. (See Tab. 1—5)

3) Five Kinds of Punctures

Miraculous Pivot(灵枢,Ling Shu) says, "In acupuncture, there are five kinds of needling corresponding to the five Zang-organs". The five kinds of needling refer to the corresponding relationship between the five Zang-organs(the lung,heart,liver,spleen and kidney) and the five constituents (the skin, vessels, muscle, tenden and bone). The five kinds of needling are also called "five Zang-organ needlings"

(1) Extremely Shallow Puncture: Extremely shallow puncture means inserting the needle superficially and withdrawing it swiftly,just like pulling out the soft hairs on the body,so that the muscles are not injured. It is used for treating pulmonary tuberculosis because skin is the manifestation of the lung. Since the needle is inserted very shallow and only half of the usual depth, it is also called semi-puncture. The main function of this technique is to dispel the pathogenic factors in the superficies of the body. Since the lung is in charge of the skin,this kind of puncture is related to the organ of the lung. In the clinic,it is applicable to treat lung diseases such as fever,cough and asthma due to invasion of the superficies by wind-pathogens. In addition,it is also used to treat some skin diseases, infantile diarrhea and indigestion. At present, a skin needle is often used when this kind of needling is conducted.

(2) Leopard-Spot Puncture: Leopard-spot puncture means piercing small blood vessels around the affected area so as to evacuate the stagnated blood. It is applicable for heart diseases due to obstruction of the meridians. In this technique, take the acupoint as the center and then, puncture scatteredly around the area to cause bleeding. It is so called because the punctured spots on the body look like leopard-spots. This technique belongs to the type of shallow puncture with blood-letting and is relevant to treat disorders of the heart which is in charge of the blood circulation. In the clinic,it is mostly used to treat diseases such as swelling and pain due to heat. It is also

applicable to treat numbness of the muscles and skin. Currently the plum-blosson needle pricking technique with heavy tapping, or scattered needling technique with the three-edged needle, is often used instead of this method.

Tab. 1—5   Table of Twelve Methods of Needlings

Twelve needlings	Needling techniques	Indications
Paired needling	Puncturing obliquely the painful area of the chest and the corresponding one on the back with one needle each	Visceral diseases, especially precordial pain
Trigger needling	Puncturing the painful area, retaining the needle until another painful trigger point is found; then withdrawing the needle and puncturing the second point	Pains which is not localized in one definite area
Lateral needling	Puncturing one side of the painful muscle, lifting, thrusting, twirling, or shaking the needlle anteriorly and posteriorly, right and left.	Spasm and pain of muscles
Triple needling	Puncturing the center of the affected part with one needle and both sides with two other needles respectively.	Affection of relatively small and deep area caused by cold
Centro-square needling	Puncturing superficially the center of the affected part with one needle and another four ones around it in a square shape. (Multiple superficial needling)	Affection of a relatively widespread and superficial area caused by cold
Perpendicular needling	Lifting the skin and puncturing subcutaneously. (Transvese puncture, subcutaneous puncture)	Affection of a relative shallow area caused by cold
Deep and perpendicular needling	Thrusting and lifting the needle perpendicularly and deeply; as few points as possible are selected.	Disease with excessive qi and heat
Short thrust needling	Inserting the needle directly to the bone area with slight shaking.	Rheumatism involving the bone
Superficial needling	Puncturing shallowly lateral to the affected part. (Oblique and shallow puncture)	Muscular spasm due to cold
Yin needling	Puncturing simultaneously the points of both lateral sides of the meridian of Foot-shaoyin.	Syncope caused by cold
Proximal needling	Puncturing the affected part vertically and laterally with one needle each.	Stubbon arthralgia
Repeated shallow needling	Repeatedly inserting and withdrawing the needle vertically and superficially, puncturing shallow with multiple needles to cause bleeding.	Carbuncles

(3) Joint Puncture: Joint puncture means puncturing the muscular fascia, or the tendon of the muscles around the joints of the limbs to avoid hemorrhage. It is used mainly to treat rheumatoid arthritis, because tendons are the manifestations of the liver. This technique requires the needle to be inserted at the muscle tendon around the joints of the four limbs. This is because

the extremities of the muscles all lie near the joints, so it is termed "joint puncture". It is also called "Yuan puncture" or "Qi puncture". Since the needling site of this technique is the tendon which is controlled by the liver, this technique is relevant to the liver. In the clinic it is applicable for muscular rheumatism and dyskinesia. But since the needle is inserted comparatively deep, attention should be paid to avoid the bleeding due to accidental puncture of blood vessels.

(4) Muscle Puncture (Multi-Direction Needling): Muscle puncture means puncturing the muscle of the affected region directly with the needle going obliquely right and left, just like the claws of a chicken, indicated in treating numbness and pain of muscles which are the manifestations of the spleen. This technique requires to insert the needle at the area where the muscle is thick, then withdraw it to the superficial part and manipulate it obliquely right and left like the claws of a chicken. This needling is done at the boundary between the muscles which is dominated by the spleen, so this technique is relevant to the spleen. In the clinic, it is applicable to treat numbness, spasm and pain of muscles, dyskinesia and muscular injury. (See Fig. 1—13)

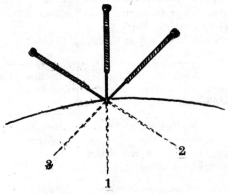

Fig. 1—13   The Muscle Puncture
(Multi-Direation Puncture)

(5) Deep Vertical Puncture: Deep vertical puncture means thrusting the needle deeply to the bone and lifting it perpendicularly to treat osteal pain because bones are the manifestation of the kidney. This technique requires the needle to be inserted directly to the bone, then withdrawn perpendicularly. Since this method needs the needle to reach the bone which is controlled by the kidney, it is revelant for the kidney and can be used to treat rheumatism involving the bone.

The contents of the five kinds of needling may be summarized as follows. (See Tab. 1—6)

The techniques of acupuncture recorded in *Yellow Emperor's Internal Classic* (内经, Nei Jing) may be classified as the following. (See Tab. 1—7).

Tab. 1—6   Table for Five Sorts of Needlings

Five punctures	Needling techniques	Indicated body constituents	Corresponding five Zang-organ
Extremely shallow puncture	Puncturing superficially with the needle withdrawn swiftly, just like pulling out soft hair on the body	Skin	Lung
Leopard-spot Puncture	Scattered puncturing with blood evacuated	Blood vessels	Heart
Joint (Fascial) puncture	Puncturing the muscular fascia or insertion of the muscle around the joints	Tendon	Liver

Five punctures	Needling techniques	Indicated body constituents	Corresponding five Zang-organ
Muscle puncture (Multi-direction puncture)	Puncturing the muscle with the needle inserted obliquely right and left, like the claws of a chicken	Muscle	Spleen
Deep and verticle puncture	Thrusting the needle deeply to the bone and withdrawing it vertically	Bone	Kidney

Blood-pricking type {

Collateral needling—Puncturing the subcutaneous small blood vessels (One of the nine types of needling)

Repeated shallow needling—Inserting and withdrawing the needle vertically. Puncturing shallow with multiple needles to cause bleeding; Applicable to carbuncle. (One of the twelve methods of needling)

Leopard-spot puncture—Puncturing the small blood vessels with multiple needles to cause blood-letting; treating swelling and pain due to heat. (One of five kinds of needlings)

Drainage needling—Incising the affected part with a sword-shaped needle to evacuate the pus and blood; Applicable to discharge of pus. (One of the nine types of puncture)

Multi-needle puncture type {

Paired needling—Puncturing obliquely the painful area of the chest and the corresponding one on the back with one needle each; used for treating cardiac obstruction. (One of the twelve methods of needling)

Triple needling—Puncturing the center of the affected part with one needle and both sides with another two needles respectively; Applicable to the affection of relatively small and deep area caused by cold. (One of the twelve methods of needling)

Centro-square needling—Puncturing superficially the center of the affected part with one needle and another four around it in a square shape; Used for treating affection of a relative widespread and superficial area caused by cold. (One of the twelve methods of needling)

Proximal needling—Puncturing the affected part vertically and laterally with one needle each; applicable to stubborn arthralgia. (One of the twelve methods of needling)

Trigger needling—After the withdrawal, the needle is used again to puncture another painful trigger point; used to treat pains which are not localized in one definite area. (One of the twelve methods of needling)

Crossing puncture type {

Opposing needling—Puncturing the points on the meridians (One of the nine types of needling)

Contralateral needling—Puncturing the points on the collaterals

} Treating the diseases of the right side of the body by needling the acupoints of the left side and vice versa.

Other type {

Cauterized needling—Puncturing the affected area with a red-hot needle; Applicable to arthralgia due to cold (One of the nine types of needlings)

Tab. 1—7 Table for Classifications of Techniques of Acupuncture Recorded in *Yellow Emperor's Internal Classic*(内经，Nei Jing)

Ⅳ. Common Procedures of Acupuncture Therapy

Acu-technique administered with filiform needles is the foundation of other various needling methods and also the part which is difficult to master in the learning process of acupuncture manipulation. The whole process of the administration of filiform needles may be summarized in six steps: ① The insertion of the needle. ② The attainment of needling sensation. ③ The direction of the transmission of the needling sensation. ④ The reinforcing and reducing manoeuvres. ⑤ The retaining of the needle. And ⑥The withdrawal of the needle. Besides, in order to obtain a better acu-esthesia below the needle and strengthen the effect of directing the transmission of acu-esthesia, it is necessary to wait for, or induce, the needling sensation to link up the intermittent needle sensation and dredge the meridians. In the process from the insertion to the withdrawal of the needle, emphasis has been placed from the ancient times until now on "the full attention of the acupuncturist" and "spiritual concentration of the patient" so as to help to achieve the desired curative result.

The procedure of acupuncture with a filiform needle is demonstrated as follows. (See Fig. 1 —14)

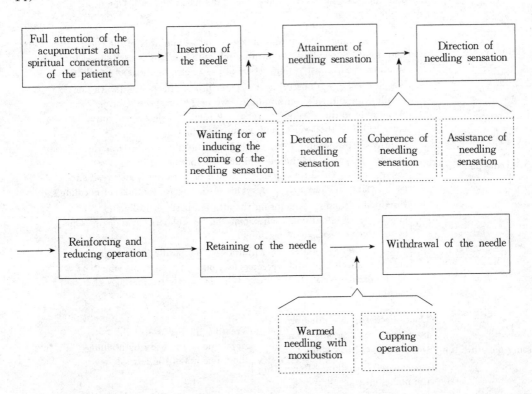

Fig. 1—14 Acupuncture Procedures of Filiform Needle

For every procedure, each step has its own special rules and different manoeuvres which are required to be mastered comprehensively by constant practice to attain the purpose of handling the needle freely and skillfully, enabling the whole needling process to be conducted consistently. Detailed information will be presented in Chapter Two of this book.

V. Prevention and Management of Possible Accidents in Acupuncture Therapy

In acupuncture administration, sometimes there may occur some unexpected accidents because of the clinician's improper manipulation, negligence in respecting the contraindications, carelessness, incompetency or poor quality of the needle appliance.

1. Acupuncture Syncope (Needling Fainting)

Acu-syncope refers to the patient fainting during the course of acupuncture treatment, which generally can be avoided if the clinician pays attention to the status of the patient.

(1) Causes: Weak and debilitated patient with undue nervousness or mental anxiety, needling after exhaustion, hunger, excessive perspiration, diarrhea or hemorrhage, improper posture of the patient or violent manipulation of the clinician and hot or suffocating weather. Such fainting often occurs when the needle is inserted, or during the retention of the needle, or at the moment when the patient rises to his or her feet as soon as the needle is withdrawn from the body.

(2) Manifestations: The patient suddenly presents symptoms of mental fatigue, vertigo, dizziness, pale complexion, nausea, hyperhidrosis, choking sensation in the chest, palpitations, shortness of breath and a deep and fine pulse. In severe cases, symptoms of shock may appear as cold limbs, coma, urinary and fecal incontinence, fainting and indistinct pulse.

(3) Management: If syncope occurs, stop needling immediately, have the patient lie on his back and withdraw all the needles out of the body. Meanwhile, attention should be paid to keep the patient's body warm. Generally, if it is a mild case, the patient can recover lying on his back for a while and drinking some warm boiled water or sugar water. For severe cases, the recovery of the patient can be obtained by puncturing the points Shuigou (DU 26), Neiguan (PC 6) and Zusanli (ST 36), or administering moxibustion on the Baihui (DU 20), Guanyuan (RN 4) and Qihai (RN 6) points.

If the patient remains unconscious with short and faint breathing and thin and feeble pulse after the above treatment, other emergency measures should be taken.

(4) Prevention: For a patient who is receiving needling treatment for the first time or who is excessively nervous about and afraid of the needling, or has a weak and debilitated body, it is necessary that the clinician explain the procedure to dispel the misunderstandings of the patient about acupuncture. Simultaneously, the clinician should help the patient choose a comfortable and convenient posture, preferably the recumbent posture. The needling points selected should be as few as possible and the manipulation mild. If the patient is hungry, tired or thirsty, he or she should be asked to take some food, have a short rest or drink some water prior to the insertion of the needles; or the puncture should be temporarily stopped. The clinician should concentrate on the patient, constantly taking notice of the patient's complexion and facial expressions or other external manifestations and inquire about the patient's feelings during acupuncture. Once signs of syncope such as pale complexion, trance and oppressive sensation in the chest occurs, early measures should be taken to avoid the occurrence of syncope.

2. Sticking of the Needle

In the course of the manipulation, or after retention of the needle, the clinician sometimes will find the inserted needle is blocked and difficult to manipulate, i. e. impossible to be rotated, lifted, thrusted or withdrawn, while the patient feels severe pain in the needling area. This situation is known as "stuck needle".

(1) Causes: Local strong muscular contraction(local myospasm) due to excessive nervousness of the patient when the needle is inserted, or the winding of muscle fibres around the needle due to excessive rotation of the needle in one direction only.

(2) Manifestations: The needle is in the body surface. The clinician feels the needle is stuck and difficult or impossible to rotate, lift, thrust or withdraw. If the clinician tries to do so, the patient may have unbearable pain in the punctured area.

(3) Management: If the case is caused by local excessive muscular contraction due to the patient's mental stress, it can be relieved by the following measures: ① Slight prolongation of the needle retention. ②Gentle massage around the point. ③ Tapping the needle tail or having one or two additional needles inserted close to the stuck needle to reduce the muscle spasm. If the case was caused by improper needle manipulation, or one-way needle rotation, it may be removed by rotating the needle backwards and twirling it right and left slightly to relax the muscle fibres and restore them to their normal condition.

(4) Prevention: For the patient who receives needling treatment for the first time or who has mental stress about acupuncture, explanatory work should be done to dispel tension and misunderstandings about needling. In order to prevent the occurrence of the muscle fibres winding around the needle, the clinician should try to avoid one-way twirling, unduly large angle of twisting and improper fast twirling when manupulating the needles.

3. **Bending of the Needle**

It refers to the bending of the needle during insertion or after the needle is inserted into the body.

(1) Causes: Unskilled or inaccurate manipulation of the clinician during insertion of the needle, undue exertion of strength(over-violent manipulation), the needle touching on hard tissues of the body, the patient's change of posture during the course of puncturing, or , accidental movement of the needle handle by foreign objects; or the unsuccessful management of a stuck needle. If the acupoint lies close to the joints of the body, or the patient is liable to muscle spasm, the spontaneous movement of the patient, when punctured, may also bring about the bending of the inserted needle.

(2) Manifestations: Bending of the inserted needle causes a change of the original direction and angle of the handle of the needle when it is inserted or retained. As a result, there occurs a difficulty in lifting, thrusting, twirling and withdrawing the needle, and a sensation of pain in the patient as well.

(3) Management: In the case of a bent needle, discontinue the manipulations (lifting, thrusting or twirling) immediately. If the needle is slightly bent, try to withdraw it by slowly following the course of the bend. If the bending angle of the needle is unduly large, the needle should be withdrawn in the direction of the curvature of the bent needle. If it is due to the shifting of the position by the patient, first, help the patient restore his or her body slowly to the original position, and then, after the local muscles are relaxed, gradually withdraw the needle. Be sure to avoid withdrawing or pulling the needle out suddenly and violently in case the needle is broken in the body.

(4) Prevention: The clinician should have a good command over the inserting manoeuvre and be proficient at needle insertion. The force exerted on the needle by the fingers should be mild and even. The patient should take an appropriate and comfortable posture. During the course of the needle retention, the patient should be asked not to shift the position casually. Take care to protect the puncturing area and avoid the accidental movement of the needle handle by foreign objects.

4. **Breaking of the Needle**

This refers to a situation where the needle is broken within the body when the needling is being conducted.

(1) Causes: Poor quality of the needle, corrosion of the needle shaft or root and failure to check it before insertion, full insertion of the needle into the human body, violent lifting, thrusting and twirling of the needle which can cause strong contraction of the muscles, casual shifting of the position by the patient in the course of needling retention, accidental movement of the needle handle by foreign objects, failure to deal with a stuck or bent needle timely and correctly, or sudden increase of intensity when electro-needling is being administered.

(2) Manifestations: When the needle is being manipulated or is going to be withdrawn, it is found broken. In this case, the broken needle may leave a certain length outside the skin or may be entirely embedded inside the body.

(3) Management: The clinician should keep calm and ask the patient not to be panic and shift his or her original position so as to prevent the distal broken fragment of the needle from sinking deeper into the muscles. In case the end of the broken fragment of the needle is above the skin, use the fingers or tweezers to pull the needle out. If the broken end of the needle is at the level of the skin vertically, press the skin around the needling hole with the thumb and index finger of the left hand to make the broken end more exposed. Then, pull it out with the forceps. In case the broken fragment end is completely under the skin surface or in the deep muscles, it must be localized by X-ray and removed by surgery.

(4) Prevention: Check or inspect the quality of the needle prior to puncture, use only a smooth and flexible needle with a fixed firm root, and dispose those which don't conform to quality requirements. Avoid violent and strong needling manipulations. When manipulating or retaining the needle, the clinician should ask the patient not to casually shift posture or position. When puncturing is done, the needle shaft should not be inserted entirely into the acupoint, some part of the needle body should be left(0. 2—0. 3 cun, i. e. 6—9 mm)above the skin so as to be able to remove the fragment of the broken needle out easily in case the needle gets broken. For cases with a bent or stuck needle, timely and correct management should be carried out. When electro-needling is used, the output intensity button of the instrument should be first placed in the "0" position before gradually increasing the intensity.

5. **Hematoma**

This refers to the subcutaneous bleeding and swelling pain occurring in the punctured area when acupuncture treatment is given.

(1) Causes: The impairment of the skin and muscles, or the injury of blood vessels due to the minute hooks or divided tip of the needle.

(2) Manifestations: Local swelling distention and pain after withdrawal of the needle with local red-purplish skin.

(3) Management: For minute amounts of subcutaneous bleeding with a small patch of hematoma, no treatment is needed and it can subside by itself. If the local swelling and pain are comparatively severe and cause an inability to move about, it is necessary to place a cold compress on the affected area. After the bleeding stops, apply a hot compress or mildly rub the local area to promote the dissipation of stagnated blood.

(4) Prevention: Check or examine the needle carefully, become familiar with the anatomy of the human body and try to avoid pricking the blood vessels. Needling manipulation should be mild and dexterous. For the points in the vicinity of the eyes, special attention should be paid to prevent the occurrence of hematoma. For area where bleeding easily takes place, apply heavy compression with cotton balls for a comparatively long time right after the needle is withdrawn.

6. Infection

This refers to the acute inflammatory reaction occurring in the needling area or the whole body after acupuncture is administered.

(1) Causes: The entry of pathogens into the body due to failure of strict sterilization of the needle, of the needling area and of the clinician's hands; or the infection of the puncture hole after the needle is withdrawn from the points.

(2) Manifestations: It may present different clinical manifestations due to different affected sites and various types of pathogens.

(3) Management: Generally, it is dealt with in the same way as the management for acute infection.

(4) Prevention: According to the rules described in the Section of Preparation Before Acupuncture, sterilization must be carried out before acupuncture. In addition, for the patient who has received acupuncture treatment for a long period, acupuncture should not be conducted repeatedly at the same site. Alternative points should be used so as to avoid the impairment of the tissues and difficulty in their regeneration, thus, decreasing the chances of infection.

7. Residual Sensation

This refers to the lingering needling sensation at the insertion point felt by the patient following the withdrawal of the needle. Appropriate residual needling sensation is a normal reaction of acupuncture.

(1) Causes: Mostly due to intense stimulation resulting from the clinician's heavy manipulation.

(2) Manifestations: Lingering soreness, pain, distention, heaviness, numbness and other uncomfortable sensations in the locality after withdrawal of the needle.

(3) Management: For a mild case, the sensation may immediately vanish or take a favourable turn when the locality is pressed up and down with fingers. For the serious case, besides the above local pressing method, moxa roll moxibustion may also be applied to dissolve the residual sensation.

(4) Prevention: Try not to manipulate the needle heavily or violently. In addition, after the withdrawal of the needle, up and down finger massage on the locality can prevent the occurrence of residual sensation.

8. Pricking Injury of Zang-Organs(Viscera)

(1) Traumatic Pneumothorax

If the points are needled unduly deep when acupuncture is conducted in the region of the chest, back or around the clavicle, the lung may be punctured, bringing about traumatic pneumothorax which is marked by pectoralgia, chest distress and palpatation. In severe cases, dyspnea, tachycardia cyanosis, perspiration and a fall in blood pressure may appear. During check-up, percussion and ausculation will show that the intercostal space of the chest on the affected side widens, the trachea is displaced towards the healthy side of the chest, the percussion note on the diseased side of the chest increases, the border of cardial dullness narrows and vesicular breath sounds on the diseased side largely decrease or even disappear as compared with the healthy side of the chest. With a chest X-ray examination, further diagnosis may be made. There are some cases which don't assume any obvious abnormal phenomena at the time acupuncture is administered. It is several hours later that abnormal symptoms of chest pain and dyspnea may gradually appear, to which special attention should be paid.

In order to effectively prevent the occurrence of pneumothorax, the clinician must concentrate on the insertion of the needle, help the patient choose a proper and comfortable position and strictly obey the rules of correct direction, angle and depth of puncture. Also, the lifting and thrusting amplitude of the needle should not be too great and the duration of needle retaining should not be too long. Once pneumothorax occurs, the patient must be sent to a hospital, observed closely and given immediate medical aid.

(2) Piercing Injury of the Heart, Liver, Spleen, Kidney and Other Internal Organs

In the course of acupuncture treatment, if the heart, liver, spleen, kidney and other corresponding areas of these organs are punctured perpendicularly and unduly deep, severe consquences may result, especially for patients who suffer cardiomegaly or hepatosplenomegaly, so special attention should be paid to them.

If the liver or spleen is accidently injured, bringing about bleeding, the patient may feel a pain in the hepatic or splenic regions, or radiating pain to the back. If the bleeding is serious and cannot be arrested, the patient may be accompanied with signs of peritoneal irritation such as abdominal pain, contraction of abdominal muscles, and tenderness or rebound tenderness of the abdomen. Injury of the kidney may lead to lumbago, tenderness or percussion pain in the renal region, accompanied with hematuria. If the bleeding is profuse, shock and low blood pressure may occur.

Once the internal organs are injured, in mild cases, the damage can heal on their own if the patient rests in bed. If suspicious signs of bleeding appear, close observation should be taken to notice the degree of the bleeding and change of the blood pressure. Also hemostat or a local cold compress should be administered to stop bleeding. In cases of serious injury accompanied by shock, emergency treatment must be given.

During acupuncture treatment, all other organs such as gallbladder, urinary bladder, stomach, intestines have the possibility of injury, esp. in cases of gallbladder enlargement, uroschesis and intestinal adhesion. If the large blood vessels are punctured, massive hemorrhage may occur.

In order to prevent the internal organs from being injured when points on the abdominal region are needled, attention should be paid while percussing the corresponding organs. For patients who suffer from hepatomegaly, gallbladder enlargement, splenomegaly and kidney enlargement, acupuncture should not be done at the points where the internal organs lie interiorly. Or they may be punctured superficially so as not to injure the organs. For the patient with a full stomach or urinary bladder or corpulent, the acupoints on the region of corresponding organs can not be needled deeply and heavily.

(3) Piercing Injury of the Brain and Spinal Cord

When the points Yamen(DU 15), Fengfu(DU 16), Fengchi(GB 20) and Jiaji(Ex−B 2) are punctured incorrectly, the medullary bulb may be injured, causing serious consequences. If the points of the Du meridian above the first lumbar vetebra are punctured too deeply, the spinal cord may be injured and the patient may have an electrifying sensation which radiates to the distal ends of the four extremities. In addition, heavy manipulation can also bring about a residual sensation. Thus, when these points are needled, the clinician should try to concentrate on needling, constantly observe the different needling response and be careful to avoid unneccesary lifting and thrusting manipulations. If the manipulation is unduly heavy, which causes excessive stimulation, temporary paralysis of the four limbs may result. If the blood vessels are stabbed, bleeding and hematoma may appear. Once the brain or spinal cord is pricked, the patient should rest and be kept under observation. Usually, after some time, the injury can heal on its own accord. If symptoms of headache, nausea, vomiting, or even coma appear, emergency treatment should be given immediately.

(4) Piercing Injury of the Nerve Trunk

When the points in the area of nerve trunks and nerve roots are punctured, an electric-like sensation may occur. If they are punctured repeatedly, the nerve tissues may be injured, bringing about dysfunction of sensation or movement, or the phenomena of burning pain and reflex muscular spasm or contracture. For the mildly-impaired case, the patient may return to normal by administering massage. For the severe case, they should be treated with drugs containing vitamin-B. In order to prevent the nerve trunk from being injured, when points in the areas of nerve trunks and roots are needled, intensive stimulation should be avoided. Simultaneously, the other corresponding points should be alternatively used in a planned way.

VI. Precautions in Acupuncture Therapy

This section, including the needling contraindications, refers to the points which the clinicians should pay attention to in acupuncture treatment to prevent the occurrence of mistakes and accidents.

Patients who are suffering from malnutrition, hunger, exhaustion and excessive mental stress are considered unfit for immediate puncture. Debilitated patients with deficiency of both qi and blood should try to choose a recumbent posture when punctured and the clinician's manipulation should not be too violent.

For women in the first three months of pregnancy, acupoints on the lower abdomen should not be punctured. For the woman who is beyond the first three months, the points on the abdomen and lumbosacral region are also contraindicated. In addition, during the pregnancy, the points Sanyinjiao(SP 6), Hegu(LI 4), Kunlun(BL 60) and Zhiyin(BL 67) must not be needled. The woman who is menstruating usually should not be punctured unless for menstrual disease. Before the closure of an infant's fontanel, the points on the vertex can't be punctured. Moreover, because of children's uncooperation during acupuncture treatment, long-time static retention of the needle is usually avoided.

When punctured, the needle should be kept away from the blood vessels to prevent the occurrence of bleeding except the case which requires blood-letting therapy. It is contraindicated to apply puncture to the patient who is vulnerable to spontaneous bleeding or who has incessant bleeding(poor blood coagulation) after an injury.

For the patient who has infections, ulcers, scar or tumors, needling can not be administered directly on the local affected areas. Be careful to prevent important organs from being pierced.

When puncturing, the clinician must master, according to the anatomic structure of important organs, the angle and depth of the needle insertion and avoid lifting, thrusting and twirling the needle in a large amplitude or retaining the needle for a comparatively long time so as to prevent the occurrence of medical accidents. *Plain Question*(素问, Su Wen) says, "The Zang-organs are the vital parts of the body which cannot but be detected". *Plain Question*(素问, Su Wen) also points out that, "if any point on the chest and abdomen is punctured, the needle must be kept away from the five Zang-organs." So special attention should be paid to the following: When the points around the eyes are punctured, appropriate angle and depth of needle insertion is the first consideration. Also, the lifting, thrusting and twirling of the needle in a large amplitude or the long-time retention of the needle should be avoided so as to prevent any piercing injury of the eye ball or occurrence of bleeding in this area.

The points on the both sides of the 11th thoracic vertebrae, the ones above the 8th intercostal in the midaxillary line and the ones above the 6th intercostal in the midclaicular line are not to be punctured perpendicularly or deeply so the heart and lungs are not injured, esp. for the patients who suffer from pulmonary emphysema and cardiomegaly.

The points in both the costal and renal region should not be punctured perpendicularly or deeply so as to avoid injuring the liver, spleen and kidney, especially for the patient with hepatomegaly or splenomegaly.

For the patient who suffers from uroschesis, if the lower abdomen needs puncturing, appropriate angle and depth of needle insertion should be taken so the urinary bladder and other organs are injured, causing unexpected consequences.

When the points on the nape and spinal vertebrae need puncturing, appropriate angle, direction and depth of needle insertion should also be taken.

VII. **Practising Methods of Needling Skills**

Since the body of the filiform needle is slender and flexible, if the clinician applies inadequate finger force and performs incorrect needling manoeuvres, it will be hard to insert the needle or administer different needling manipulations at will. Practice of both finger force and manipulation is basic in raising the standard of needling technique and is also essential for ensuring the smooth administration of acupuncture in clinical treatment, avoiding pain in the patient and increasing therapeutic efficacy.

1. **Practice of the Finger Force**

During the administration of acupuncture, the left hand is usually used as the pressing hand (i. e. the hand which is applied to press hard on the skin adjacent to the acupoint to help the insertion of needle), while the right hand is used as the needle-holding hand, (i. e. the hand holding the handle of the needle). Comparatively speaking, the right hand is more important than the left in needling. In acupuncture treatment, desired therapeutic result depends mainly on the appropriate manipulations and the exerting force of both hands. The exerting force is chiefly embodied in the thumb, index and middle fingers. The force exerted in both needling manipulation and transmission of the needling sensation rests in the fingers. However a dexterous and painless insertion of the needle requires the converging force from the palm, wrist, arm or even the whole body. Only with this kind of force, can the needle be inserted into the body dexterously and painlessly. If a learner wants to be a competent acupuncturist and achieve satisfactory results in the clinic, he or she must keep practising to have the thumb, index and middle fingers proficient in any needling manoeuvre. The exerting finger force has a close relationship with the needling manipulation. To learn acupuncture and moxibustion, it is necessary to practice finger force. There are many methods to practice it, among which the paper-pad and cotton-ball needling methods are the most common.

Finger force practice can be first conducted on a paper pad or cotton ball (The paper pad is made by having soft paper folded into a cake-shaped pad which is 8cm long, 5cm wide and 2cm thick, wrapped tight with a thread for use. The cotton ball is made by wrapping some cotton within gauze and binding it tight with a thread. The size should be 6-7cm in diameter). For beginners, it is better to practice perpendicular needling first with short filiform needles on the paper pad or cotton ball. In doing so, the needle should be kept upright as far as possible as if holding a Chinese writing brush, holding the body of the needle vertically to the paper pad or cotton ball. Just before the needle tip touches (reaches) the pad or the ball, finger force is gradually exerted to make the needle enter the pad or ball. Keep doing so until the needle can be smoothly, dexterously and rapidly inserted into the pad or ball. (See Fig. 1—15, 1—16). Using the same method of vertical needling, continue practising the lifting, thrusting, twirling and other essential needling manoeuvres.

In acupuncture treatment, the key to needling manipulation is finger force. But the so-called finger force does not only refer to strength, but a kind of "qi" force. Many acupuncturists in ancient times believed in the sayings that, "Building up the body and regulating the breathing (training respiration) before manipulating the needle" and "The administration of all the techniques of acupuncture must firstly rely on the acupuncturist's vitality. " These were recorded in the book The *Yellow Emperor's Internal Classic*(内经,Nei Jing).

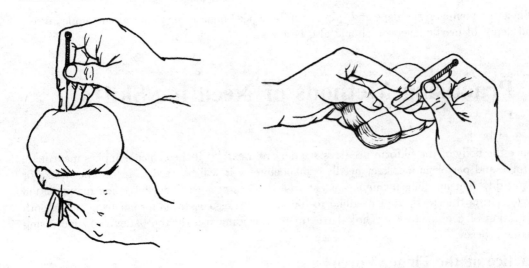

Fig. 1—15 **The Practice of the finger**
Force on the Cotton Ball

Fig. 1—16 **The Practice of the Finger**
Force on the Paper-Pad

Besides good finger force, some palm force is also necessary in needling manipulation. Therefore, many well-known acupuncturists attach importance to the practice of palm force with a view to increasing the strength of the metacarpophalangeal joints. This helps one easily gain the needling sensation and make the conduction of needling sensation along the meridian more obvious, ensuring a better curative effect.

Sometimes because of the administration of some complex acupuncture techniques such as heat-producing needling, or cold-producing needling, the acupuncturist needs to take a sitting posture to ensure the even and exact operation of finger force. Sitting steadily for a long period of time is another skill for the clinician to practice.

2. Practice of the Common Manipulations

Practising perpendicular insertion of the needle on a paper pad or cotton ball, other commonly used elementary needling manipulations can also be conducted on the pad and ball.

(1) Practicing Quick Puncturing

Use the thumb and index finger of the left hand to hold the paper pad or cotton ball and the right hand to hold the needle. Insert the needle vertically and quickly into the supposed point on the pad or ball. Keep doing so repeatedly to master needle insertion.

(2) Practicing Twirling-Rotating Puncturing

Use the thumb, index and middle fingers of the right hand to hold the needle. After the needle is inserted, use the thumb and index fingers to hold the handle and twist it at the original spot clockwise with the thumb moving forwards and the index finger backwards and counterclockwise with the thumb moving backwards and index finger forwards. The twisting angle should be even and the manipulation should be dexterous and consistent in speed. It is generally accepted that twirling 150—200 times per minute can reach the requirement (the needle shaft should rotate at over 150—200 turns per minute).

(3) Practicing Lifting-Thrusting Puncturing

Use the thumb, index and middle fingers of the right hand to hold the needle. After insertion of the needle, lift and thrust the needle repeatedly and moderately at the insertion point. When doing so, the needle should reach the desired and appropriate depth. Moreover, the needle body should always be kept vertically throughout the whole process.

(4) Practicing Repeated Lift-Thrusting Puncturing

This is a quick needling method with repeated lifting and thrusting at the inserted spot in a small range, just like a bird pecking food, so it is also known as bird-peck needling. When practising, use the thumb, index and middle fingers of the right hand to hold the needle. After the needle is inserted, fix the middle finger vertically beside the needle, lift and thrust the needle repeatedly either with the thumb and index fingers, or with the vibration of wrist joint of the right hand. When doing so, the needle should be vertical and lifted at the same needling hole in the same direction and consistantly at the same depth.

To gain proficiency in finger force and the different manipulations mentioned above, the comprehensive practice of various manipulations can be conducted on a paper pad and cotton ball.

3. Self-Needling Test

After having acquired a good grasp of finger force and needling techniques on the paper pad or cotton ball, the student may select some points on his or her own body where the muscle is thick enough to do self-needling. If conditions permit, students can do the test on each other. By self-needling, the clinician can realize the toughness of the skin, the degree of the strength exerted when the needle is inserted and the varied sensations after the insertion of the needle. Generally when self-needling is done, the points of Hegu(LI 4), Quchi(LI 11) and Zusanli (ST 36) are often chosen for use since they have an obvious needling sensation and are comparatively safe.

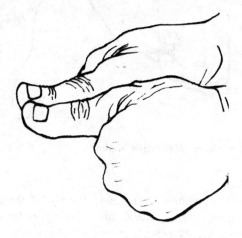

Fig. 1—17 **The Double-Thumb Fingers Meditation Method**

Appendix: Supplementary Practicing Methods of Needling Skills

1) Other Practicing Methods of the Finger Force

(1) Double Thumb-Fingers Meditation Method

Take a standing position near the table, breathe in air and direct it to Dantian. Lift and stretch both arms forwards, then bend the body forward with the thumbs of both hands pressed at the edge of a table(See Fig. 1—17). Concentrate the mind on Dantian and spontaneously feel the qi in Dantian running upwards to both shoulders, then, through the arms, elbows and wrists down to the thumb tips. If the clinician feels it difficult to stick to the thumb exercise, the index fingers may be used instead of the thumbs to practice at the edge of the table. (See Fig. 1—18). Keep doing so alternatively several times. In the beginning, practice may last 5 minutes once or twice a day. Later, the practicing time may increase to 15 minutes. As a rule, initial results can be obtained in about 15 weeks.

(2) Three-Finger Confrontation Method

Close the middle and index fingers of one hand tightly, forming a hook shape; then, have the thumb tip press the middle and index fingers, making the tips of the three fingers touch closely the part between the thumb and the index finger, forming a round shape. Then knock violently at something hard several times with great strength. Keep practicing as long as you can. (See Fig. 1—19).

(3) Wood-Cone Clamping Method

Hold two small wood-cones with the thumbs, index and middle fingers of both hands and roll them repeatedly with the fingers. The cones should be 3 cun long, 1 cun thick with the root thick and the tip thin. Keep practicing it as long as possible every day and good results can be obtained in six months. (See Fig. 1—20)

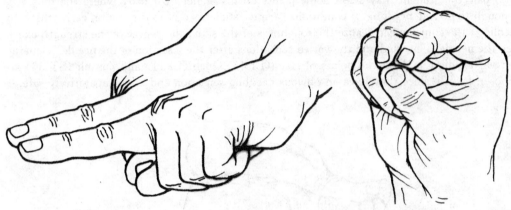

Fig. 1—18   **The Double-Index Fingers Meditation Method**   Fig. 1—19   **The Three-Finger Confrontation Method**

(4) Thread-Twisting Method

This method does not need any material. Just keep the tips of the thumb, index and middle fingers touching each other with part of the thumb and index finger forming a triangle. After the tips of the three fingers are closed tight, exert the strength of the whole body on the finger tips. Do the thread-twisting motion with the thumb rotating forward and then backwards several times. Keep practicing it as long as possible.

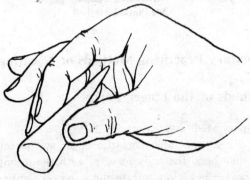

Fig. 1—20   **The Wood-Cone Clamping Method**

2)Palm-Moving and Qi-Training Method

This method is a type of health-cultivation method in Qigong practice. However, with the gradual increase of palm-moving force, it can assist in the manipulation of acupuncture and enhance the needling curative effect. For instance, when the "reinforcing" and "reducing" methods are administered, if the palm and finger forces are sufficient and strong, the"rotating"and"scraping"techniques can be applied flexibly.

The main contents of this method include "heaviness", "lightness", "inclination", "tendency", "stretch","flexion", "rotation" and "parallel", which are known as "The Eight Palm-Moving Techniques". The manipulation process is as follows:

When the palm is pushed forward, the force above the cubital articulation should be exerted heavily, while the force below it should be exerted lightly. When the palm is withdrawn backwards, the force below the cubital articulation should be heavy and the force above it should be light. In doing so, whether the palm is pushed or pulled, and force is exerted heavily or lightly, the practitioner must elevate the primordial qi, tranquilize the mind and concentrate the attention on the palms. When the palm is pushed outwards, the inclined strength should be exerted from the upper part of the elbow(from elbow joint to shoulder joint)and when the palm is withdrawn, the strength should be exerted from the lower part of the elbow(from the elbow joint to the fingers of the hand). When the palm is pushed outwards, the arm is also stretched, which helps spread the qi of the whole body. When the palm is withdrawn, the arm is simultaneously bent, which helps converge the qi of the whole body. The repeated movements of palm pushing and withdrawing constitite the rotating motions. The push and withdrawal of the palms requires the upper part of the body to be erect and the arms to be parallel to the shoulder. The detailed movements are related as follows:

(1) Take a standing posture with both hands drooping naturally(See Fig. 1—21), the centers of the two palms facing interior at the lateral sides of the thighs. Remove distracting thoughts, concentrate the mind and close the mouth naturally with the tongue touching the palate. After regulating the breathing evenly, slightly inhale the Qi from the soles of both Yongquan points(KI 1) up to the Dantian area. Then, after a slow expiration, "elevate" the Qi from Dantian to the subdiaphragmatic area and finally "conduct" it to the shoulder extremity of the right arm.

Place the feet 30—40cm apart with the knees flexed slightly and the upper part of the body in a slight squatting posture. Simultaneously, lift the bent right arm up to the shoulder level with the fingers stretching, palm facing downwards and the thumb pointing to the center of the upper part of the chest, where the point Tiantu(RN 22) lies. Flex the left arm with the palm stretched and press the hand on the lateral side of the lumbo-iliac region with the four fingers pointing forwards and the thumb pointing to the right side(See Fig. 1—22). Then, stretch the right arm laterally outwards. This is called "palm pushing"(See Fig. 1 —23). When the palm is pushed, the force exerted above the elbow should be heavy and below the elbow it should be light. After the palm is pushed, the arm should be flexed immediately and the palm will returns to the center of the upper part of the chest. This is called palm withdrawal (See Fig. 1—24). When the palm is withdrawn, the force exerted below the elbow should be heavy and above it should be light. Continue doing the pushing and withdrawing movements ten times, then stop and restore the body to its original position. (See Fig. 1—25).

(2) After completing the pushing and withdrawing movements of the right hand and regulating the respiration, do the same movement with the left hand. The method is similar to those in the right hand though there is a difference in the left and right forms(See Fig. 1—26,1—27, 1—28,1—29). Do the movements of the right and left hand alternatively. At first, ten minutes are enough for practice.

(3) After acquiring proficiency in doing the alternative left and right hand movements,

practice double palm movements. This method is as follows:

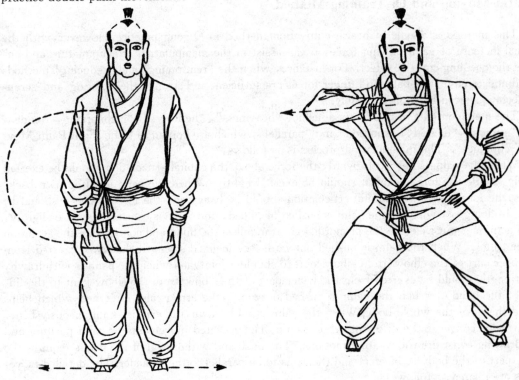

Fig. 1—21   **The Beginning Posture**
of Standing

Fig. 1—22   **The Beginning Posture**
with the Right Hand

Take a standing posture, "lift" the Qi from the soles of the feet up to Dantian. Then "elevate" the Qi to the subdiaphragmatic area and "conduct" it along the arms to both shoulders. At the same time, spread the feet apart, raise the two arms outwards with the palms facing downwards, bend the arms to the chest with the two thumbs pressed at the center of the chest directly under the two clavicles, the other eight fingers of the two hands approximated with each other and paralleled to the shoulders (See Fig. 1—30). Then, push both the right and left palms outward simultaneously (stretch both the left and right arms outward simultaneously). Afterwards, do the withdrawn movements (See Fig. 1—31, 1—32). Continue doing so for about ten times; then, restore the body to its original standing posture (See Fig. 1—33). Generally the double-palm movements are done for ten times. However, if no fatigue sensation is felt in the upper limbs or whole body, more movements can be added.

3) Sitting-Training Method

When complicated needling techniques such as heat-producing and cool-producing needling are administered, the clinician is required to keep the body erect and stable. Sitting-training has proved to be an effective practice for clinician. The detailed method is as follows:

Regulate the breathing and concentrate the mind, sit erect with the chest thrown out, shoulders squared and the back straight. Cross the legs with the right leg over the left, the dorsums of both hands resting on the knees and the eyes on the nose. Expirate and inspirate slowly from shallow to deep by first "exhaling" the turbid qi from the chest and then "inhaling" fresh air. When inhaling the air, have the "inhaled" Qi go through the chest and then into the Dantian. At

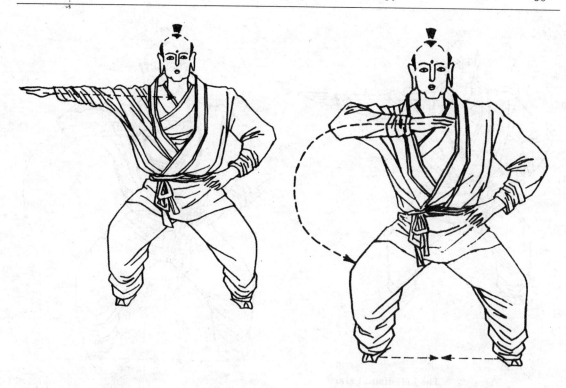

Fig. 1—23 **The Right-Hand Palm Pushing Posture**

Fig. 1—24 **The Right-Hand Palm Withdrawing Posture**

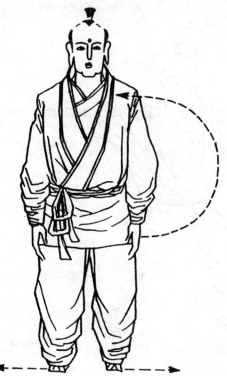

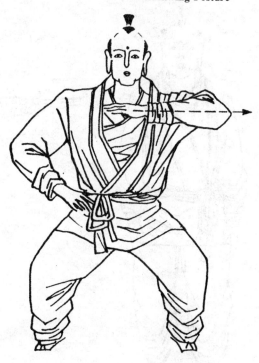

Fig. 1—25 **The Closing Posture**

Fig. 1—26 **The Beginning Posture with the Left Hand**

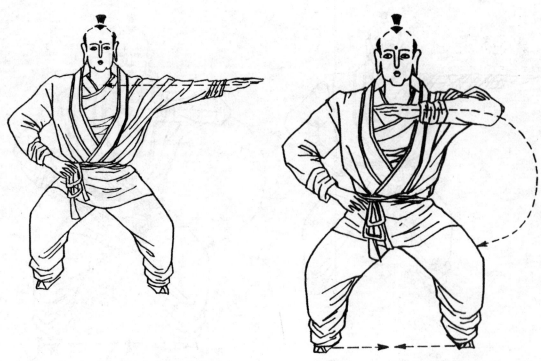

Fig. 1—27   **The Left-Hand Palm Pushing Posture**

Fig. 1—28   **The Left-Hand Palm Withdrawing Posture**

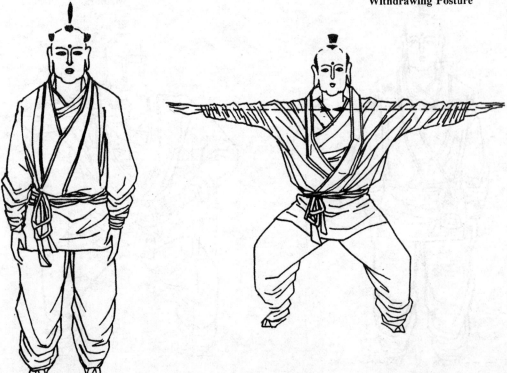

Fig. 1—29   **The Closing Posture**

Fig. 1—30   **The Both-Hand Palm Pushing Posture**

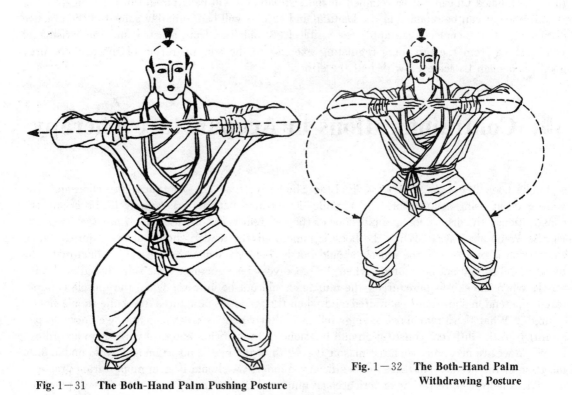

Fig. 1－31   **The Both-Hand Palm Pushing Posture**

Fig. 1－32   **The Both-Hand Palm Withdrawing Posture**

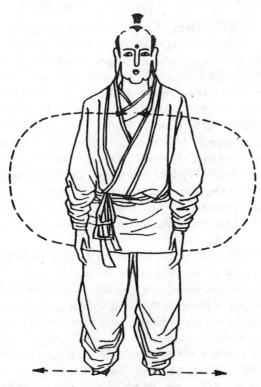

Fig. 1－33   **The Closing Posture**

first, the inhaled Qi can not be retained in the Dantian and will be expired. But if sitting-training is continued, it can be retained in the Dantian and success will be ultimately gained in the practice of Qigong . If the clinician can apply the visible force obtained from practice and the invisible qi (air) gained from the breathing-regulating exercise to the administration of the acupuncture, good results can be achieved with half the effort.

VIII. Contraindications in Acupuncture Therapy

The book *Miraculous Pivot* (灵枢, Ling Shu) says that "In old times, the clinicians who were good at using acupuncture and moxibustion treated patients accordingly by observing the constitutions, the disposition and physique of the different types of patients". *Plain Questions* (素问, Su Wen) also says, "When the body is punctured, the tendon should not be injured; when the tendon is punctured, the muscle should not be injured; when the muscle is punctured, the blood vessel should not be injured; when the blood vessel is punctured, the skin should not be injured; when the skin is punctured, the muscle should not be injured; when the muscle is punctured, the tendon should not be injured; and when the tendon is punctured, the bone should not be injured". What these two above sayings tell us is that when we treat patients, we ought to pay attention to the different constitution and physique of the patients and deal with them accordingly. When we are needling, we must master the depth of the needle insertion and avoid undue deep insertion of the needle. All these are benificial reminders we should bear in mind during practice. Thus, it is helpful to relate the experiences accumulated by the ancestors in their clinical practice.

1. Contraindicated Regions

Plain Questions (素问, Su Wen) says, "The body has its vital parts which cannot but be detected. " This means that each internal organ of the body is a vital part. The clinician should know and be familar with the location of its organ. When a needle is administered, great attention should be paid to it. If needling is done too deep, bad consequences can occur. For instance, if the point Quepen(ST 12) is punctured too deeply, the lung will be injured and dysfunction of lung-qi will occur, causing cough with dyspnea. *Plain Questions* (素问, Su Wen) says, "If the chest is punctured unduly deep, the lung will be injured, leading to dyspnea and rapid respiration. If the heart is punctured, the patient may die in one day···If the lower abdomen is unduly punctured, the urinary bladder can be stabbed and urine will accidently leak out, causing the lower abdomen to be filled and distend. If the head is unduly punctured, the brain can be damaged and the patient may die immediately. " All the above indicate that if important organs such as the lung, heart, liver, spleen, brain and spinal cord are injured, life-threatening accidents may be brought about. Thus, on these regions where important internal organs lie, deep needling is absolutely forbidden.

It is also pointed out that in areas where important blood vessels lie points should be punctured cautiously, esp. for the sites where the arteries lie. For instance, *Plain Question* (素问, Su Wen) says, "If the artery on the foot instep is injured, blood will flow endlessly, causing death. If the artery in the posterior region of the knee is damaged, the patient may collapse because of depletion of the spirit. If the iliac veins are punctured, the blood will not bleed out of the body, but cause an internal hematoma. If the femoral artery is injured, endless hemorrhage will be the result, causing death", "If the Taiyin blood vessels on the arms are punctured, much blood will be lost, causing immediate death. " These all show that if important vessels are injured, uncontrolled hemorrhage, or even death will occur. In addition, there are some records which say that if the sublingual artery is unduly punctured, hemorrhage will take place consistently, causing aphasia. If the facial veins are punctured, blindness may accidently be caused. If the veins distributed over the feet are punctured, the blood will not bleed out, but cause blood swelling. If the knee-cap is punctured and fluid is discharged, a limp will be the result. If the joints are punctured and fluid is discharged, disability of limbs in stretch and flexion may be brought about. All these experiences the ancient people accumulated in the past should not be ignored. We should attach great importance to them.

2. Contraindicated Acupoints

The contraindicated acupoints basically rest on the contraindicated regions mentioned above. Many medical documents of past ages had records to this context though there are discrepancies in them. In *Great Compendium of Acupuncture and Moxibustion*(针灸大成, Zhen Jiu Da Chen), acupoints such as Naohu(DU 17), Xinhui(DU 22), Shenting(DU 24), Yuzhen(BL 9), Luoque (BL 8), Chengling(GB 18), Luxi(SJ 19), Jiaosun(SJ 20), Chengqi(ST 1), Shendao(DU 11), Lingtai(DU 10), Danzhong(RN 17), Shuifen(RN 9), Shenque(RN 8), Huiyang(BL 35), Henggu (KI 11), Qichong(ST 30), Qimen(LR 14), Chengjin(BL 56), Shousanli(LI 10), Sanyangluo(SJ 8), Qingling(HT 2) and Ruzhong(ST 17) are listed as ones which can not be punctured. But, in fact, from the viewpoint of modern clinical medicine, except for Shenque(RN 8) and Ruzhong(ST 17) which are absolutely incapable of being needled, all of them can be punctured.

It is also necessary to note that all the points on the nape of the neck, chest, and back can not be deeply punctured with long needles and carelessly lifted or thrusted with thick needles. When the points Qichong (ST 30), Qimen (LR 14), Renying (ST 9), Jingqu (LU 8), Chongyang(ST 42), which lie near blood vessels are to be punctured, the needle should be kept off the vessels. The fontanell of an infant can not be punctured. The lumbo-abdominal region and the points Hegu (LI 4), Sanyinjiao(SP 6), Quepen(ST 12) and Jianjing(GB 21) in pregnant woman should be punctured with caution. In a word, the key in avoiding accidents is to master the manipulation, direction and depth of the needling.

3. Contraindication According to the Patient's Condition

Miraculous Pivot(灵枢, Ling Shu) says, "There are five kinds of exhaustions which are characterized respectively by excessive emaciation(first exhaustion), massive hemorrhage(second exhaustion), profuse perspiration(third exhaustion), severe diarrhea(fourth exhaustion) and severe loss of blood during delivery(fifth exhaustion). The patient with any of the five kinds of exhaustions must not be punctured with reducing manipulations". The five kinds of exhaustions mentioned above are all serious conditions caused by excessive consumption of qi, blood and body fluid. Because of this, the reducing method is contraindicated. *Miraculous Pivot*(灵枢, Ling Shu) also says, "Insufficiency of both physique and qi will result in deficiency of pathological qi, thus causing deficiency of both Yin qi and Yang qi, so acupuncture can't be conducted. If puncture is done, excessive deficiency may occur, which brings about exhaustion of both Yin and Yang, consumption of blood and qi, deficiency of the five Zang-organs and withered tendons, bones and marrow. As a result, the old will die and the strong can't make a recovery." The above shows that the patient who manifests an emaciated body marked by pallor complexion, shortness of breath and faint pulse should be contraindicated for acupuncture. Before needling, the clinician must observe the physique and complexion of the patient and be sure not to aggravate the deficiency. *Miraculous Pivot*(灵枢, Ling Shu) also points out that the patient who suffers from the five exhaustion syndromes should not be punctured. All of these experiences provide useful information for our clinical practice.

4. Provisional Contraindications

Plain Questions(素问, Su Wen) says that, "No acupuncture is done on drunken persons or the person who suffers from dysfunction of qi; no acupuncture is done on a person in rage or the one who may suffer from reversed flow of qi; no acupuncture is done on the person in fatigue, in satiety or in great hunger…, no acupuncture is done on the person who is frightened. " *Miraculous Pivot*(灵枢, Ling Shu) also says that, "Acupuncture has many contraindications. The person who has just eaten his fill can't be punctured, and the one who has just been punctured can't be fed; The drunken can't be punctured while the person who has just been punctured can not drink. The person who is angry can't be punctured while the one who has just been punctured should not get angry. The person who is in fatigue can't be punctured and the one who has just been punctured should not get fatigue. The person who is in satiety can't be punctured and the one who has just been punctured should not eat his fill. The person who is in hunger can't be punctured and the one who has just been punctured should not be hungry. The person who is thirsty can't be punctured and the one who has just been punctured should not be thirsty; Extreme terror(fight) and rage lead to disorder of qi, so puncture must be done after the patient calms down. For the patient who is carried to see the acupuncturist, puncture is done after the patient has taken a rest on a bed for the amount of time it takes for one to have a meal. And for the one who comes to visit the acupuncturist on foot, the puncture is done after he or she has taken a rest for the amount of time it takes for one to walk 5km. For the patient who has any of the 12 kinds of contraindications, since his or her four systems (Ying, Wei, blood and Qi)are in disorder, which causes disturbances in the pulse and qi and if the patient is punctured …, qi will be lost. " All the above shows that when needling is administered, the patient's daily life and dietetic condition before and after acupuncture treatment are also important and can't be ignored by the clinician.

Chapter Two

Manipulations of Filiform Needle in Acupuncture Therapy

This chapter discusses the main filiform needling techniques which include the different methods of manipulation such as insertion of the needle, attainment of needling sensation, transmission of needling sensation, reinforcing and reducing manoevres and withdrawal of the needle. Besides, the needle-holding method, the vitality-controlling method and point-through-point method which are related directly to the filiform needle are also dealt with comprehensively.

I. Methods for Controlling the Vitality

This method, also called the vitality-regulating method, concerns geratly with the therapeutic results of the treatment. The Book *Plain Questions* (素问, Su Wen) says that, "The real essence of needling must be based on controlling the mental activity." The book *Miraculous Pivot* (灵枢, Ling Shu) also says that, "Each kind of acupuncture manipulation must be based on mental activity", which shows the importance of this method. The vitality controlling method refers to the technique of inducing the needling sensation by means of regulating the patient's mental activities and concentrating the mind of the acupuncturist. It can be divided into two aspects: the concentration of the acupuncturist's mind and regulation of the patient's mental activity. The so-called "concentration of the acupunturist's mind" means that the acupuncturist should, before and after needle insertion, concentrate the energy and pay full attention to the patient, observing the patient's spirit and complexion and experiencing the puncturing response under the needle tip. He should do just as the *Plain Questions* (素问, Su Wen) says that, "The one who operates the acupuncture should feel as if he is standing beside the abyss, or grasp the needle like holding a tiger's tail. Pay attention to nothing but the patient, without looking at any other place… " So

Miraculous Pivot(灵枢, Ling Shu) says that, "The vitality manifests distinctively. If the patient suffers from mental disturbances, the acupuncturist should examine the patient's qi and blood and give acupuncture treatment according to the condition, which brings about no complications. " Guoyu (郭玉), a famous acupuncturist in the East Han Dynasty once said "One's attention should be embodied in the cooperation and harmony between the mind and the hands. "

The so-called "regulation of the patient's mental activity" means to make the patient's distracted spirit return and remove the thoughts of panic and anxiety during needling. Calm the patient by explaining the aim of the treatment to enable the patient to receive the acupuncture treatment in a good psychological state. *Songs of Secret on Acupuncture and Moxibustion*(标幽赋, Biao You Fu) says, "All who administer acupunture should insert the needle after the patient feels at ease; and even after the needle is inserted, calmness of the mind is needed to induce the needle sensation. There should be no needle insertion until the patient feels at rest. " *Plain Questions*(素问, Su Wen) also says, "Calm the patient's spirit, give an explanation, then operate the acupuncture timely. "These two quotations emphasize the importance of regulating the patient's mental activity. In clinical application, this vitality-controlling method is often conducted in two steps: ① Regulating the mind before inserting the needle, and ② Concentrating on the needle tip after inserting the the needle.

Regulation of the mind before needle insertion refers to adjusting the mental conditions of both the acupuncturist and patient, enabling the acupuncturist to concentrate his or her mind on the administration of the needle and the patient to feel at ease and peace during the procedure. Therefore, the *Great Compendium on Acupuncture and Moxibustion* (针灸大成, Zhen Jiu Da Cheng,) says, "The so-called spirit-calming is just to regulate or stablize the mind of the acupuncturist and the patient. No needling is done when the mind is not at rest. "

Concentration on the needle tip after needle insertion means that after obtaining the needling sensation, the acupuncturist is still required to pay attention to the inserted needle tip so as to keep the needling response from being dispersed; Thus, *Plain Questions*(素问, Su Wen) says, "If the qi arrives, try to keep it and make sure not to lose it. The needling sensation, no matter how deep it appears and how far it moves, depends on the acupuncturist's vitality and spirit. " *Miraculous Pivot* (灵枢, Ling Shu) also says, "When puncturing, one should concentrate his energy and draw attention to the needle. " All the above indicates that only when the mind is focused on the inserted needle, will the curative effect be enhanced.

This vitality-controlling method begins with the regulation of the mind of both the acupunctnrist and patient. Then, after the needle is inserted into the body, it requires the acupuncturist to continue paying attention to the needle until the needle is withdrawn. This means that control of the vitality must be present throughout the whole needling process. If the acupuncturist wants to make the essence of vitality reach the fingers and wrist which he is using to hold and manipulate the needle, he should practise some Qigong(气功) and Taiji(太极拳) to ensure that vitality reaches a high state.

Ⅱ. Methods of Holding the Needle

In acupuncture manipulation, the clinician usually uses both hands. The hand holding and manipulating the needle is called "the puncturing-hand" and the one which is used to assist in the needle insertion by pressing on the area close to the acupoint is called "the pressing-hand". In the clinic, most of the clinicians use the right hand to hold the needle and the left to facilitate the insertion of the needle. Thus, the right hand is known as the "puncturing hand" and the left as the "pressing hand".

The book *Miraculous Pivot*(灵枢, Ling Shu) says, "The right hand is in charge of holding and pushing the needle and the left hand is in charge of fixing the needle. " The book *Classic on Medical Problems*(难经,Nan Jing) says," The one who knows about the needle manipulations pays attention to the left hand,and the one who does not know the needle manipulation only pays attention to the right hand. " The book *Songs of Secret on Acupuncture and Moxibustion*(标幽 赋,Biao You Fu) also says, "Pressing the acupoint area longer and more heavily with the left hand causes qi(needling sensation) to spread easily; inserting the needle slowly and gently with the right hand induces no pain. " These three quotations all state the importance of the coordination of both hands during the puncturing process. The puncturing hand plays the role of handling the needle,making the needle tip pass quickly through the skin and into the body. It also conducts various manipulations such as twirling, rotating, lifting and thrusting. The pressing hand plays the role of fixing the location of a point, minimizing the possible pain sensation to the patient during the needle insertion, supporting the shaft of the needle and avoiding the occurrence of rocking and bending of the needle so that the insertion of the needle can be done easily. In addition,the pressing hand can be used to strengthen the needle sensation, promote the needling sensation and regulate the needling response.

Needle-holding method refers to the way that the clinician handles the needle. *Miraculous Pivot*(灵枢,Ling Shu) says, "As far as the needle-holding skill is concerned,the needle is required to be held firmly. " The commonly used needle-holding methods are:

1. Holding the Needle with Two Fingers

Use the thumb and index finger of the puncturing hand to grasp the handle of the needle. (See Fig. 2—1) This is suitable for puncturing with short needles.

2. Holding the Needle with Three Fingers

Grasp the needle by the thumb of the puncturing hand on one side and the index and middle fingers on the other side of the needle. (See Fig. 2—2) This is suitable for puncturing with relatively long needles.

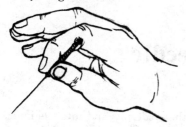
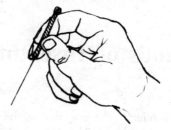

Fig. 2—1   **Holding the Needle**
with Two Fingers

Fig. 2—2   **Holding the Needle with**
Three Fingers

3. Holding the Needle Shaft with Fingers

Hold the lower part of the shaft of the needle, which is bound with a sterilized cotton ball, with the thumb and index finger of the puncturing hand, aim the tip at the acupoint and quickly insert the needle into the skin. (See Fig. 2—3)

4. Holding the Needle with Both Hands

Grasp the handle of the needle with the thumb, index and middle fingers of the puncturing hand and hold the needle tip closely with the thumb and index fingers of the pressing hand(See Fig. 2—4). This is suitable for puncturing with a long needle or an elongated needle. The coop-

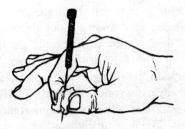

Fig. 2－3   Needle-Body-Holding Method

eration between both hands can ensure the needle is inserted easily and prevent a bent needle. In addition, there are several other needle-holding methods, but no matter which method is adopted, the clinician should keep a straight posture and calm the mind and hold the needle firmly and puncture the area accurately.

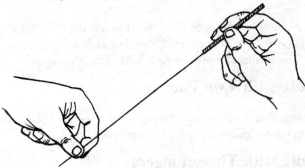

Fig. 2－4   Holding the Needle with Both hands

Ⅲ. Methods of Inserting the Needle

These methods refer to the insertion of the needle through the epidermis and into the inner skin or subcutaneous tissue. Command over these methods is directly related to the clinical effect. *Great Compendium on Acupuncture and Moxibustion*(针灸大成, Zhen Jiu Da Cheng) says, "When inserting the needle, both the patient and the acupuncturist should keep the breath even and the mind at rest. The acupuncturist should not be hasty, but should locate the acupoints carefully." What it explains is that when inserting the needle, both the doctor and patient should have a peaceful and stable frame of mind. Only in this way, pain caused by puncturing can be reduced or even eliminated.

The insertion of the needle can be classified into two kinds: i. e. insertion with one hand and insertion with both hands.

1. Insertion of the Needle with Single Hand

In the clinic, the most commonly used method is to grasp the handle of the needle with the thumb and index finger of the puncturing hand, with the medial side of middle finger against the lower portion of the shaft and the tip of the middle finger close to the acupoint. Insert the needle into the acupoint to the designated depth by downward pressure of both the thumb and the index finger and the flexing movement of the middle finger. This method is used mostly while puncturing with short needles. (See Fig. 2—5)

2. Insertion of the Needle with Both Hands

1) Inserting the Needle with Aid of the Finger of the Pressing Hand

Press on the acupoint with the nail of the thumb, index finger or the middle finger of the left hand (pressing hand). Hold the needle with the right hand and insert the needle into the skin close to the edge of the nail of the finger of the left hand. Usually, this method is applied for short needles. (See Fig. 2—6)

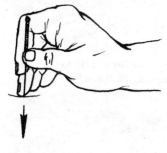

Fig. 2—5　Inserting the Needle
with One Hand

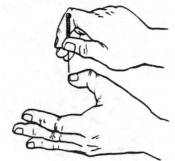

Fig. 2—6　Inserting the Needle with the Aid of
the Finger of the Pressing Hand

2) Gripping and Inserting the Needle

Grip the lower portion of the needle shaft with the thumb and index fingers of the left hand which have been sterilized. Hold the handle of the needle with the right hand like holding a Chinese writing brush and place it directly over the surface of the acupoint, then quickly insert the needle into the skin with pressure exerted with two hands which act in cooperation. Usually this method is used for inserting long needles. (See Fig. 2—7)

3) Inserting the Needle by Pinching up the Skin

Pinch up the skin around the acupoint with the thumb and index fingers of the left hand. Hold the needle with the right hand and insert the needle into the pinched skin. Usually this method is applied during insertion on the areas where the skin and muscle are flabby and thin. (See Fig. 2—8)

4) Inserting the Needle by Stretching the Skin

Put the thumb and index finger, or the index and middle fingers, on the skin where the acupoint is located. Separate the two fingers to stretch the skin tightly, then insert the needle with the right hand. This technique is suitable for puncturing areas where the skin is loose or with wrinkles. (See Fig. 2—9)

In addition, there are other methods which require devices to insert the needle, e. g. the insertion the needle with the help of a guiding tube, but at the present time they are not widely used in China.

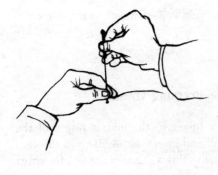

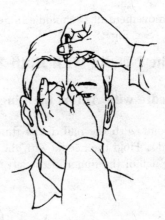

Fig. 2—7   **Inserting the Needle by Gripping it**

Fig. 2—8   **Inserting the Needle by Pinching up the Skin**

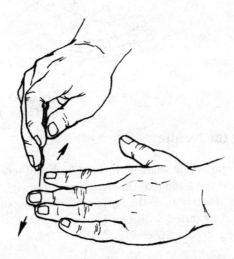

Fig. 2—9   **Insertion of the Needle by Stretching the Skin**

IV. Methods of Manipulating the Needle

This method refers to the manipulation of the needle after insertion. The purpose of this manipulation is to induce needling sensation, direct the transmission of the sensation and reinforce or reduce the sensation by lifting, thrusting, twirling, rotating the needle or changing the angle of the needling in the acupoint. The basic needle manipulations are lifting-thrusting, twirling and rotating.

1. Lifting and Thrusting Manipulation

This refers to the lifting up and thrusting down of the needle during acupuncture. After the needle is inserted to a certain depth, do repeated lifting and thrusting movements, thereby making the needle move from the deep to the superficial. (See Fig. 2 –10). The amplitude and frequency of this movement should vary with the patient's physical constitution, pathological condition and also with the location of the acupoint. However, comparatively large amplitude and high frequency should be avoided. In general, large amplitude and rapid frequency result in strong stimulation and a small amplitude and slow frequency result in gentle stimulation.

2. Twirling and Rotating Manipulation

This refers to twirling or rotating the handle of the needle clockwise and counter lockwise alternately after the needle has been inserted into the specific depth required (See Fig. 2–11). The angle and frequency of the twirling or rotating movement should vary with the patient's physical constitution, pathological condition and location of the acupoint. A large angle and high frequency rotation results in strong stimulation while a small angle and low frequency rotation results in weak stimulation. In general, the angle of twirling or rotating should be below 360°. In addition, the clinician should not twirl the needle in only one direction, otherwise the needle body easily gets tangled with the muscle fibers, bringing about local pain in the patient.

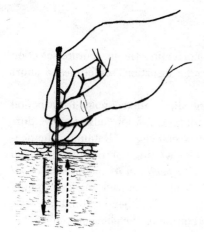
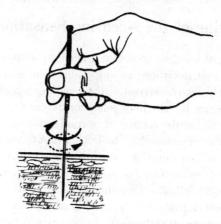

Fig. 2–10 Lifting and Thrusting Method   **Fig. 2–11 Twirling and Rotating Method**

V. Manipulations of Attaining, Awaiting and Inducing Needling Sensation

1. Attaining of the Needling Sensation

This refers to the heavy and tense reaction felt by the clinician and the local sensation of soreness, numbness, heaviness and distension experienced by the patient after the insertion of the needle. In acupuncture treatment, only after the needling sensation is attained and appropriate manipulation of reinforcing-reducing is administered, can a satisfactory curative effect be obtained. *Songs of Secret on Acupuncture and Moxibustion*(标幽赋, Biao You Fu) says, "The light, slippery and sluggish feeling indicates the failure of attainment of the needling sensation , while tight, astringent and strong analgesia suggests the approach of needling sensation. When the needling sensation comes, there may appear a tight and floating sensation like a fish eating bait on a fishhook. When the needling sensation fails to come, a hollow feeling occurs as if someone has entered into an empty house. " This vividly describes the characteristics of the needling sensation felt by the patient and the clinician. It is suggested that when administering acupuncture, the clinician must concentrate his or her mind and be careful to experience the needling reaction. The judgement of whether the needling sensation is attained or not should be the first consideration.

In addition, the speed and intensity of the attainment of needling sensation are related to the condition of the patient and the needling techniques of the clinician. Failure to obtain the needling sensation has many causes which include: inaccuracy of acupoint selection, incorrect mastery of the needling angle, direction and depth, sluggishness of flow of qi due to deficiency of meridian qi and a debilitated body. If this occurs in a seriously ill patient, it usually indicates the consumption of meridian qi. What is emphasized here about needling sensation is that the pursuit of acu-asthesia should be appropriate. There is no need to obtain intense needling sensation. Undue needling sensation can, on the contrary, reduce the curative effect, or even bring about fainting or other accidents.

Sometimes, even though the needling sensation is weak and the patient does not have the obvious sensations of soreness, numbness, heaviness and distention, a curative effect can still be achieved, which is the so-called "latent sensation" in acupuncture.

2. Awaiting of the Needling Sensation

In case of a failure to obtain a needling sensation, besides correcting the inaccurate selection of acupoint and deviations in angle, direction and depth of needle insertion, sometimes, a short time is needed for the arrival of the needling sensation.

Waiting for the needling sensation refers to retaining the needle in the acupoint for a period of time to wait for the coming of normal sensation when the needling sensation fails to arrive during acupuncture treatment. The book *Plain Questions*(素问, Su Wen) says, "Retaining the needle for a long time until the needling sensation comes is just like waiting for the distinguished guest without considering the approach of the evening". *Great Compendium of Acupuncture and Moxibustion*(针灸大成, Zhen Jiu Da Cheng) also says that, "Of all the procedures in acupuncture treatment, waiting for the coming of needling sensation is the first". They both indicate that when the needling sensation fails to be attained in acupuncture treatment, the clinician can use the asthesia-awaiting method to wait for the arrival of needling sensation.

3. Inducing of the Needling Sensation

In acupuncture, when the needling sensation fails to be obtained, some manoeuvres can be applied to induce the occurrence of it. Just as *Songs of Golden Needles*(金针赋, Jin Zhen Fu) says, "If the needling-asthesia fails to attain, it is induced by massaging along the meridians with fingers…; Twirling, twisting and flicking the needle until the sensation comes". But, it should be pointed out that this kind of asthesia-inducing manoeuvre is a method adopted only in the case of failure to obtain the needling-asthesia or in the case where the needling sensation has been obtained but is inadequate after the needle is inserted correctly into the desired acupoint. However, it can also serve to strengthen the needling sensation and play a role in assisting, keeping and directing the needling sensation. The commonly used methods in inducing the sensation are of the following nine kinds:

1) Meridian-Massaging Method

After inserting a needle into an acupoint to a certain depth, press or massage the skin with fingers gently along the course of the meridian where the acupoint is located. (See Fig. 2—12) *Great Compendium of Acupuncture and Moxibustion*(针灸大成, Zhen Jiu Da Cheng) says that, "When the needle is inserted, if the needling sensation fails to attain, massage the course of the related meridian of the acupoint up and down or sideways with fingers to promote the flow of qi and blood. When the qi and blood circulates evenly, the tight and heavy sensation will naturally arrives". This method is mainly used to excite the meridian and promote the circulation of meridian-qi to have the needle sensation induced easily. This method can also be applied in directing the transmission of needling sensation.

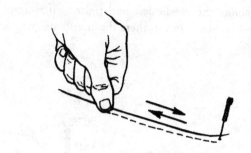

Fig. 2−12 **Meridian-Massaging Method**

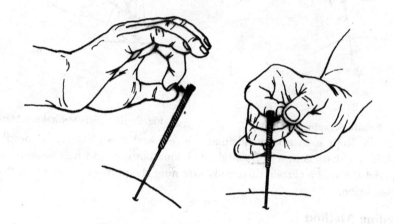

Fig. 2−13 **Needle-Flicking Method**

2) **Needle-Flicking Method**

After inserting a needle into an acupoint to a certain depth, gently flick the handle of the needle with a finger tip, causing mild vibration of the needle so as to quicken the circulation of meridian-qi. (See Fig. 2−13) Just as the *Great Compendium of Acupuncture and Moxibustion*(针灸大成, Zhen Jiu Da Cheng) says, "If flicking method is used, first flick the needle tail to wait for the arrival of needling sensation."

3) **Needle-Scraping Method**

After inserting a needle into an acupoint to a certain depth, resist the needle tail with the thumb belly and scrape the handle of the needle slightly with the nail of the index or middle finger; or resist the needle tail with the belly of the index finger and scrape the needle handle from the lower to the upper with the nail of the thumb frequently and gently. Or scrape the handle of the needle gently from lower to the upper with both thumb and index finger nails, which is known as "whirling scraping". (See Fig. 2 − 14) This scraping method is mostly used to strengthen the needling sensation and promote diffusion.

4) Needle-Shaking Method

After inserting a needle into an acupoint to a certain depth, sometimes, the needle sensation is very faint. In such cases, the needle-shaking method is often used to strengthen the weak sensation. The manipulaton is to insert the needle vertically into the body, hold the handle or body of the needle with the hand and shake the needle left and right as if ringing a bell. The purpose of doing so is to have the inserted needle vibrate, then the meridian-qi is activated. (See Fig. 2—15).

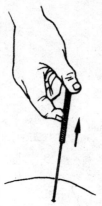
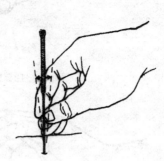

Fig. 2—14 **Needle-Scraping Method**   Fig. 2—15   **Needle-Shaking Method**

When the needle shaft is in a perpendicular position and it is shaken, the needle sensation may be enhanced. If the shaft is in a horizontal or oblique position and it is shaken, the needling sensation may spread towards a certain direction, attaining the purpose of directing the transmission of needling sensation.

5) Wing-Spreading Method

After inserting a needle into an acupoint to a certain depth, if the needling sensation is very faint, this method can be used to strengthen the sensation. The manipulation is mainly embodied in the twirling of the needle. Usually, rotate the needle with the thumb and middle finger with great amplitude, then twirl and release the needle. The movements of the needle twirling and the fingers releasing should be like the spreading wings of a flying bird. Repeat the twirling and releasing movements as if a bird spread its wings. (See Fig. 2—16). The book *Elementary Medicine* (医学入门, Yi Xue Ru Men) says, "Twirling the needle with thumb and index finger three times successively in a hand-quivering (wing-spreading) shape, which is named Fei (飞, flying)".

6) Needle-Vibrating Method

This is also termed "lifting-thrusting method". After inserting a needle into an acupoint to a certain depth, if the needling sensation is very weak although it has been induced, this method may be used to make the needling sensation stronger. The manipulation is to lift the needle gently and thrust it heavily at the inserted acupoint with less amplitude and quicker frequency. The movement should be based on the vibrations of the wrist joint. Keep the needle tip in the original point and make the inserted needle neither entered nor withdrawn, just like a bird pecking food.

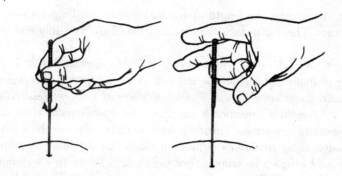

Fig. 2—16   Wing-Spreading Method

This is why it is also called " bird-pecking method. "

All the methods above can be used for the patient's different conditions. For instance, the needle-scraping and needle-flicking methods may be used for the acupoints which are unfit for the administration of great amplitude twirling; Wing-spreading and needle-vibrating methods are applicable to the points where the muscles are thick. The needle-shaking method is suitable for superficial points.

Apart from these, there are other methods which can induce the needling sensation.

7) Needle-Deepening Method

If the needling sensation fails to come after the needle is inserted into an acupoint to a certain depth, the needle can be inserted deeper to induce the needling sensation. In addition, this method also has the potential to invigorate qi and improve inspiration. In fact, this method can be considered as "lifting-thrusting" method.

8) Needle-Swinging Method

This is similar to the needling-shaking method. After the needling sensation is induced, lift the needle a bit and then, with the thumb and index finger holding the handle of the needle, repeatedly and gently swing the needle left and right to strengthen and direct the transmission of the needling sensation.

9) Needle-Thrusting-Drawing Method

First insert the needle into the earth portion of the acupoint(i. e. the deep portion of the acupoint), then, with the thumb moving backward and the index finger moving forward, withdraw (lift)the needle quickly to the heaven portion of the acupoint(i. e. the shallow portion of the acupoint)as the needle is twirled. After that, in the course of twirling the needle, thrust the needle to the earth portion again with the thumb moving forward and the index finger moving backward. When withdrawing(lifting) the needle, give milder force and when thrusting the needle, give heavier force. This method can make the needling sensation come swiftly.

Ⅵ. Manipulations of Directing the Transmission of Needling Sensation

This is also a technique for regulating circulation of Qi. It is a method to expand the area of needling sensation to and extend the length of transmission of needling-asthesia so the sensation reaches the affected part. This is, in fact, the continuation of the awaiting and inducement of the needling sensation.

The book *Great Compendium of Acupuncture and Moxibustion*(针灸大成, Zhen Jiu Da Cheng) says, "If the acupoint is far from the affected part, the first consideration is to enable the needling sensation reach the affected area." The book *Songs of Golden Needles*(金针赋, Jin Zhen Fu,) also says that, "Needling sensation runs along the meridians". Both are related to the transmission of the needling sensation. This technique actually refers to the method of controlling the propagated sensation along meridians in modern times and is one of the important factors in increasing the therapeutic efficacy in acupuncture treatment. When this technique is conducted, attention should be paid to the following: ① Determining the meridian according to the different symptoms and signs, then treating disease by dealing with the meridian and making the symptoms, meridian, and acupoints work together. ② Having an appropriate needling stimulation. Generally, it is suitable to conduct the mild or moderate stimulation; i. e. the patient has the feelings of soreness, numbness, distension and warmth without any painful sensation in the needling area, while the clinician has a bit of tight and heavy feeling upon manipulating the needle. ③. Making the direction of needle insertion accurate and the depth of the insertion appropriate to obtain the needed needling sensation. This method is also called by some people the "Inspection of needling sensation", i. e. to inspect whether the needling sensation induced is the one which is desired. ④ Taking care to seize the right time in the course of directing the transmission of the needling sensation and sustaining the sensation, and ⑤ The patient should loosen clothing and relax.

The commonly used techniques to direct the transmission of needling sensation are as follows:

1. Needle Tip-Pointing Method

This refers to the method that makes the needle tip point towards the diseased area. Just as *Catechism on Acupuncture and Moxibustion*(针灸问对, Zhen Jiu Wen Dui) says, "After the needle is inserted into the acupoint and needling sensation is induced, point the needle tip to the affected area. If the needling sensation is required to be conducted upward, the tip should be obliquely raised, and if it is required to be conducted downward, the tip should be obliquely declined. Then the needle-flicking and needle-shaking manoeuvres are used to strengthen the sensation."

2. Pressing Method

If the sensation is required to be conducted downwards after the needle sensation is induced, the pressing hand of the clinician should be used to press the area above the punctured point, which may cause the sensation to go downward when the needle-holding hand is used to manipulate the needle. On the contrary, if the needling sensation is required to be conducted upwards, the pressing hand of the clinicianer should be placed at the area below the needled acupoint. *Songs of Golden Needles*(金针赋, Jin Zhen Fu) says that, "If the anterior area of the acupoint is pressed, the needling sensation will run backwards. If the inferior area of the acupoint is pressed, the sensation will run forward." This indicates that the conducting direction of the needling sensation and the acupoint-pressing direction of the hand are opposite.

3. Needle-Down Method

This method is also termed "prone needling". After the needling sensation is induced, lift or withdraw the inserted needle to the shallow portion of the body. Incline or pull the shaft of the needle down at a certain angle and bring the tip point to the diseased part. Then administer the twirling or lifting-thrusting manipulation to conduct the needling sensation to the diseased part. (See Fig. 2—17)

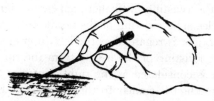

Fig. 2—17   Needle-Down Method

4. Needle-Bending Method

After inducement of the needling sensation, lift the inserted needle slightly, hold the handle with thumb and index finger and press the needle shaft sideways with the middle finger, making the needle bend like a bow. If the needling sensation is required to be spread upwards, the needle body is pressed downwards and backwards. If the sensation is required to be spread downwards, the needle body is pressed upwards and forwards. (See Fig. 2—18). This method can conduct the sensation directly to the diseased area. In order to avoid the loss of needling sensation, the administration of this method should be combined with the other pressing and twirling methods. This method is similar to the needle-down one, but the latter, in which the needle approximates to lying flat against the skin, has a smaller angle compared with the former.

5. Needle-Tapping Method

After obtaining the needling sensation by manipulating the needle, tap the needle tail vertically and frequently with the index or middle finger, making the needle move gradually deeper until it reaches a certain depth. (See Fig. 2—19)

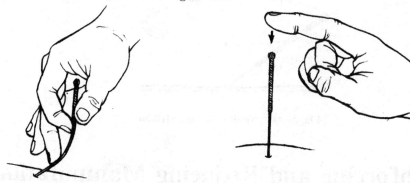

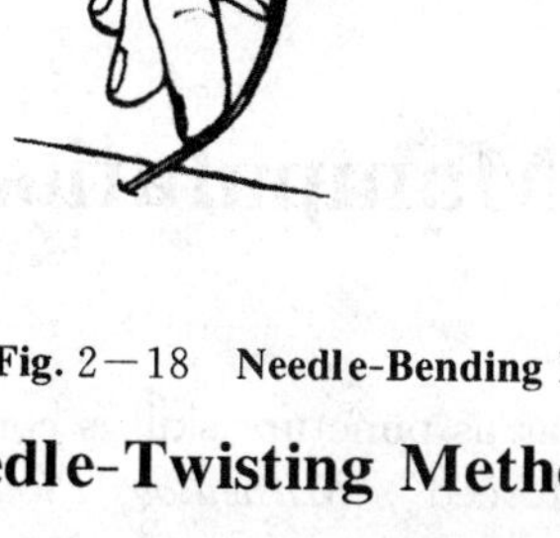

Fig. 2—18   Needle-Bending Methed

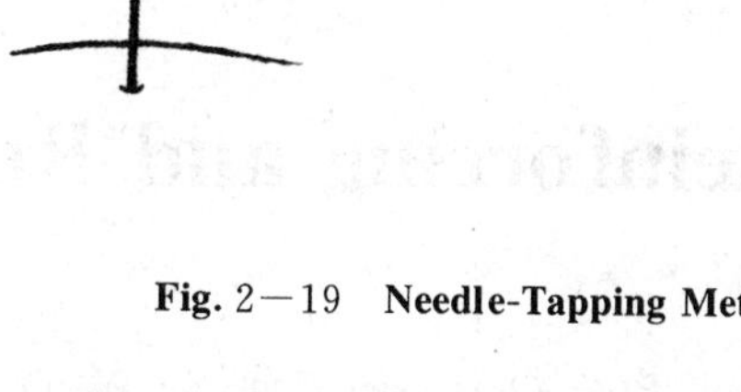

Fig. 2—19   Needle-Tapping Method

6. Needle-Twisting Method

Rotate the inserted needle in one direction, like twisting a cotton thread, to have the muscular fibres moderately wound around the needle. Make use of its drawing and pulling action to excite the meridian-qi so as to strengthen the reinforcing-reducing effect of acupuncture, pursuing the occurrence of cool or hot sensation. This is both a qi-promoting and reinforcing-reducing method.

Usually, the twisting movement begins from the cross striation of the last segment of the index finger. Twist the needle forward with the thumb up to the tip of the index finger, just like twisting a cotton thread. Stop the twisting until there appears a tight, heavy sensation as if the needle were wound by the muscles. The twisting of the needle from the cross striation of the last segment to the tip of the index finger is regarded as the left, interior and reinforcing, which often induces a hot sensation; And the twisting of the needle from the tip to the cross striation of the last segment of the index finger is considered as the right, anterior and reducing, which usually induces a cool sensation. This method is similar to the methods of heat-producing needling and cool-producing needling in many aspects.

7. Acupoint-Supplementing Method

This refers to puncturing more acupoints on the same meridian as the needled points lie to intensify a prolonged transmission of needling sensation to assist in the circulation of meridian-qi. For instance, if the acupoint Hegu(LI 4) on the Yangming meridian of the hand is selected but fail to cause its meridian-qi to go upwards to the head and face, the acupoints Quchi(LI 11) and Jianyu(LI 15) on the same meridian should be added to assist the meridian-qi in moving freely to the diseased area.

8. Needle-Circling Method

After inserting the needle into the deep part of the acupoint and obtaining the needle sensation, lift or withdraw the needle to the shallow portion of the acupoint and incline the needle shaft at an angle of 15-45 degrees to the skin surface; Then move the needle in a circle or half circle at the same angle(See Fig. 2—20). This method involves a turn of the needle in a great amplitude, so it is often used for the acupoints on the abdomen where the muscles are plentiful and flabby. Also, it can be used in the lumbodorsal region and the four extremities where the muscles are thick. When manipulating with this method, it is inadvisable to exert the force too violently and rapidly, otherwise, bending and sticking of the needle may occur, causing pain.

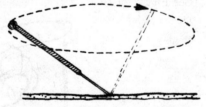

Fig. 2—20   Needle-Circling Method

VII. Reinforcing and Reducing Manipulations

The book *Plain Questions*(素问, Su Wen) says that "As far as puncture skill is concerned, the excess should be reduced and the deficiency should be reinforced". *Miraculous Pivot*(灵枢, Ling Shu) also says that, "For all who use acupuncture to treat diseases, deficiency should be reinforced; excess should be reduced; Accumulation or stagnation should be removed and excessive evil should be weakened. To treat deficient and excessive syndromes, the nine kinds of needling are the best; To reinforce or reduce, do it with acupuncture." Of which, the so-called reinforcing and reducing, in fact, are the corresponding treating principles and methods established in the light of "deficiency and excess syndrome." Acupuncturists in the past dynasties, based on the main purpose of the meridians, created many concrete deficiency-reinforcing and excess-reducing needling manipulations.

Generally speaking, the treatment with traditional Chinese medicine lies in the regulation of Yin and Yang to keep the body in a condition of "both Yin and Yang in equilibrium" so as to made the physique and body function healthy. The pharmacological treatment of Chinese medicine is achieved mainly by the exertion of the cold, heat, warm and cool natures as well as the tonifying or purgate actions of the different drugs. Acupuncture treatment, on the other hand, works through the administration of reinforcing and reducing manipulations to attain the same purpose. For instance, the needling response of "local hot sensation" and "local cool sensation" recorded in *Plain Questions* (素问, Su Wen), which later evolved into the "heat-producing needling" and "cool-producing needling" were the typical reinforcing and reducing methods. That is, through different stimulations to exert the effects of reducing excess by removing heat and reinforcing deficiency by warming Yang.

The administration of reinforcing-reducing manipulation should run through the whole process from the insertion to the withdrawal of the needle. Meanwhile, it has a direct relationship with the physical constitution and the organic state of the patient as well as the nature of cold, heat, deficiency and excess of the syndrome. The book *Miraculous Pivot* (灵枢, ling Shu) says, "Observe or examine patients' sufferings so as to find the cause of disease. Then, according to deficiency or excess, reinforce the deficiency or reduce the excess···, it's the correct treatment". This clearly points out that the reinforcing and reducing methods should be carried out according to the patient's condition and they two have an inseparable connection. Only if both are unified with each other, can the purpose of treating diseases be attained. (See Tab. 2—1)

Tab. 2—1   **Comparison of Reinforcing and Reducing Actions**

Reinforcing method	Inserting the needle during the patient's expiration	Manipulating the needle along the direction of the meridian	Inducing the needling sensation interiorly	Making the body resistance stronger
Reducing method	Withdrawing the needle during the patient's inspiration	Manipulating the needle against the direction of the meridian	Inducing the needling sensation exteriorly	Making the pathogenic qi scattered and discharged

The reinforcing and reducing manipulations can be divided into two types: the basic and the comprehensive. The basic refers to the simple reinforcing-reducing manipulation in terms of the direction of needle insertion or twirling of the needle, or in light of the speed of the needle insertion and withdrawal, or in accordance with the degree of heaviness of the needle insertion and withdrawal, or the cooperation of the needle insertion and withdrawal with the respiration. The comprehensive refers to the fact that two or more basic reinforcing-reducing manipulations are used in coordination.

In the clinic, there are 12 kinds of reinforcing-reducing manipulations, of which six kinds belong in basic manipulations and the other six belong with comprehensive manipulations. The most commonly used reinforcing-reducing manipulations are introduced as follows:

1. Reinforcing and Reducing by Lifting and Thrusting the Needle

Differentiation of reinforcing and reducing is based on whether the inserted needle is thrusted swiftly from the shallow portion of the acupoint to the deep portion, or lifted swiftly from the deep to the shallow portion.

The book *Classic on Medical Problems*（难经，Nan Jing）says，"After obtaining needling sensation，push the needle inwards to restore energy，which is known as reinforcing；then，draw the needle back to eliminate evils，which is called reducing." *Classic on medical Problems*（难经，Nan Jing）also records，"Operate reinforcing technique from Wei(shallow) part and do reducing technique from Rong(deep) part." They both indicate that after needling sensation is induced，if the needle is thrusted downwards and inwards，the manipulation is regarded as reinforcing；and，if the needle is lifted upwards and outwards，it is considered as reducing. The book *Elementary Medicine*（医学入门，Yi Xue Ru Men）emphasizes that "When operating the manipulations of lifting and thrusting needle，lift the needle quickly and thrust it slowly，just as touching ice，for reduction；And，lift the needle slowly and thrust it quickly，as being warmed by a fire，for reinforcement，" This demonstrates that on the basis of attainment of needling sensation，the heavy，swift lifting and gentle，slow thrusting of the needle from the deep portion of the acupoint to the shallow portion is the reducing；the heavy，swift thrusting and gentle，slow lifting of the inserted needle from the shallow portion of the acupoint to the deep portion is the reinforcing. (See Fig. 2—21)

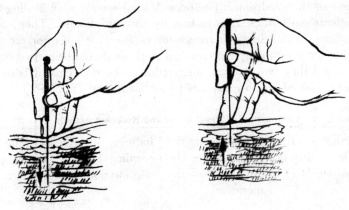

Fig. 2—21 Reinforcing and Reducing by Lifting and Thrusting the Needle

2. Reinforcing and Reducing by Twirling and Rotating the Needle

Differentiation of the reinforcing and reducing is based on whether the needle is twisted clockwise or counter-clockwise. *Miraculous Pivot*（灵枢，Ling Shu）has recordations of "holding and twirling the needle" and "slightly twirling the needle and pushing it slowly". *Plain Questions* （素问，Su Wen）says "Twisting the needle along with the respiration". The book *Guidance of Acupuncture* （针经指南，Zhen Jing Zhi Nan）states "Using the thumb and index finger to twist the needle anti-clockwise." The book *Songs of Secret on Acupuncture and Moxibustion*（标幽赋，Biao You Fu）further explains, "Puncture against the direction of meridians with the index finger twirling to the left to reduce cool. Puncture along the direction of meridians with the index finger twirling to the right to reinforce warm." All the above shows that after the presence of needling sensation，if the needle is twisted clockwise with the thumb moving forward and index finger moving backwards，this manipulation is taken as reinforcing. On the contrary，if the needle is twisted anti-clockwise with the thumb moving backwards and index finger forwards，it is taken as reducing. (Fig. 2—22)

In addition，the book *A Miraculous Classic*（神应经，Shen Ying Jing）adds that，"The

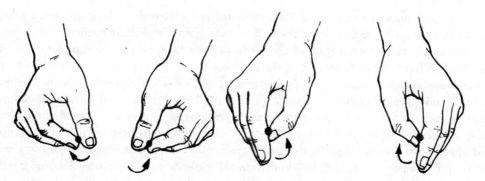

Twirling and Rotating the Needle   Twirling and Rotating the Needle
Clockwise (Reinforcing)   Anti-Clockwise (Reducing)
Fig. 2—22   **Reinforcing and Reducing by Twirling and Rotating the Needle**

twisting of the needle with the thumb moving forward is reinforcing and with the thumb moving backward is reducing. " The book *Great Compendium on Acupuncture and Moxibustion*(针灸大成,Zhen Jiu Da Cheng) also adds, "The reinforcing refers to the twisting of the needle to the left with the thumb protruding. The reducing refers to the twisting of the needle to the right with the thumb withdrawing. " It must be noted that when reinforcing manipulation is administered, more force should be exerted as the thumb moves forward and less force is exerted as the index finger moves backwards. Thus, the needle is twisted clockwise. When the reducing manipulation is administered, less force is exerted as the thumb moves backward and more force is exerted as the index finger moves forward. As a result, the needle is twisted counter-clockwise.

In the clinic, the even number 6, or the multiples of it, which is considered as Yin, is taken as the reducing; while the odd number 9, or the multiples of it, regarded as Yang, is taken as reinforcing. They are used to stipulate the frequency of needle twisting or the lifting and thrusting of the needle.

Either of the two numbers has its three different levels, i. e. the light, middle and strong, which are applied to determine the degree of reinforcing and reducing. This method is known as the nine-six reinforcing-reducing technique. (See Tab. 2—2)

Tab. 2—2   **Nine-Six Reinforcing and Reducing Technique**

	Light	Middle	Strong
Odd Number	9	$3 \times 9 = 27$ or $7 \times 7 = 49$	$9 \times 9 = 81$
Even Number	6	$3 \times 6 = 18$ or $6 \times 6 = 36$	$8 \times 8 = 64$

3. Reinforcing and Reducing by Rapid and Slow Insertion and Withdrawal of the Needle

Differentiation of reinforcing and reducing is based on the speed of insertion-withdrawal of the needle.

The book *Miraculous Pivot*(灵枢,Ling Shu) says that, "Inserting the needle slowly and withdrawing the needle quickly is for reinforcing; inserting the needle swiftly and withdrawing the needle slowly is for reducing. " This book further explains, "The so-called reinforcing by slow insertion and quick withdrawal of the needle refers to that after there appears a needling sensation, if the needle is required to be inserted further from the shallow portion of the acupoint to the deep portion, the slow insertion of the needle, compared with the speed by which the needle is withdrawn from the deep portion of the acupoint to the shallow portion, is taken as reinforcing; and the so-called reducing by quick insertion and slow withdrawal of the needle means that after the presence of needling sensation, if the needle is required to be withdrawn further from the deep portion of the acupoint to the shallow portion, the slower withdrawal of the needle, in comparison with the speed by which the needle is inserted into the deep portion of the acupoint from the shallow portion, is taken as reducing". Generally, the reinforcing method can conduct Yang-qi from the superficial to the deep and from the exterior to the interior (See Fig. 2—23). On the contrary, the reducing method may conduct the pathogenic qi from the deep to the superficial layer and from the interior to the exterior. (See Fig. 2—24)

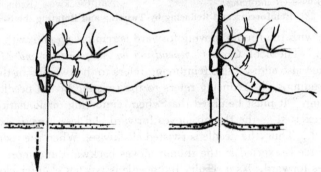

Slow Insertion   Rapid Withdrawl
Fig. 2—23   **Reinforcing by Slow Insertion**
and Rapid Withdrawal of the Needle

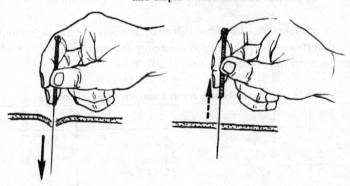

Rapid Insertion   Slow Withdrawal
Fig. 2—24   **Reducing by Rapid Insertion**
and Slow Withdrawal of the Needle

In the clinic, based on the principle mentioned above, some different formulations about reinforcing and reducing manipulations have advanced such as "first shallow, then deep", "three insertions and one withdrawal", which in fact refer to reinforcing by slow insertion and quick withdrawal and "first deep, then shallow", "one insertion and three withdrawal", which actually mean reducing by swift insertion and slow withdrawal of the needle. In addition, it is necessary to note that this kind of manipulation is closely related to the reinforcing-reducing manipulations by lifting and thrusting the needle, by deep and shallow insertion and withdrawal of the needle, and by heat-producing and cool-producing needling.

Besides, the book *Miraculous Pivot* (灵枢, Ling Shu) also explains, "The reinforcing is achieved by, apart from inserting the needle slowly and withdrawing it swiftly, quickly pressing the hole after the needle is slowly withdrawn. The reducing is achieved by, except for forceful and swift insertion and slow withdrawal of the needle, slowly pressing the hole or with the hole open after the needle is quickly withdrawn. "

Based on the explanation made by Yang Jizhou(杨继洲), the author of *Great Compendium on Acupuncture and Moxibustion*(针灸大成,Zhen Jiu Da Cheng), it may be understood that this kind of reinforcing-reducing manipulation by rapid and slow insertion and withdrawal of the needle can also be reflected in the retention and withdrawal of the needle; That is, the long-time needle retention and swift pressing of the hole after the withdrawal of the needle is for reinforcing。 On the contrary, short-time needle retention and slow pressing of the hole after the needle is withdrawn is for reducing. In the clinical treatment, these two manipulations can be integrated.

4. Reinforcing and Reducing by Puncturing Along and Against the Direction of the Meridian

Differentiation of reinforcing and reducing is based on whether the puncturing of the needle is along or against the running direction of the meridian qi.

The book *Miraculous Pivot*(灵枢,Ling Shu) says that, "By puncturing against the direction of meridian and depriving the evils,it means reduction. By needling along the direction of meridian and strengthening qi, it means reinforcement. " The book also mentions that, "For reducing, puncturing is conducted against the direction of the meridian; for reinforcing, puncturing along the direction of the meridian. Only it is known when,why and how to puncture against or along the direction of the meridian, can the qi(vital energy) be harmonized. " What these two quotations express is that the reducing refers to the insertion and operation of the needle against the running direction of the meridian and the reinforcing refers to the insertion and operation of the needle along the running direction of the meridian.

The book *Classic on Medical Problems*(难经,Nan Jing) says that, "Ying (迎)-Sui (随) means that one should know the circulation of both Ying and Wei energies and the distribution of the meridians. Then,insert the needles according to the circulating direction. " What this explains is that the regions where the Ying-qi(essential qi)and Wei-qi(defensive qi) circulate are different in depth and the direction in which the Ying-qi and Wei-qi run is changeable. So the reinforcing and reducing manipulations that are administered according to the different depth of regions,duration of flourish and weakness of the blood and qi, clockwise or counterclockwise puncturing, all belong to this kind.

The Book *Classic on Medical Problems*(难经,Nan Jing) also says that, "Puncturing against the direction of the meridian to deprive evils is to reduce the son. Needling along the direction of the meridian to invigorate qi is to reinforce the mother. " which is the reflection of this kind of manipulation imbodied in the "mother-child" reinforcing-reducing method.

From above, it may be seen that this kind of "reinforcing and reducing manipulation by puncturing along and against the direction of the meridian" includes different concepts. All the formulations mentioned above in the book *Classic Medical Problems*(难经,Nan Jing) have a wide connotation and may be regarded as reinforcing and reducing by puncturing along and against the direction of the meridian in a broader sense. The reinforcing and reducing by puncturing along and against the direction of the meridian applied in the clinic at present are mainly based on the exposition recorded in the book *Illustrated supplementary to Classic of* 81 *Medical Problems*(图注八十一难, Tu Zhu Ba Shi Yi Nan). It says that, "For reducing,adjust the needle tip pointing against the flowing direction of the meridian to meet the coming and unstrong meridian-qi so as to deprive evils,which is the so-called Ying(meeting 迎). For reinforcing,adjust the needle tip pointing along the course of the meridian-qi to follow the running and unweak meridian-qi so as to invigorate energy, which is the so-called Sui(Following 随)" The treatise recorded in *Great Compendium of Acupuncture and Moxibustion*(针灸大成,Zhen Jiu Da Cheng) explains "After getting the acupuncture feeling, make the needle tip point against the coming direction of meridi-an-qi and puncture with retreating manipulation, which is regarded as Ying(Meeting 迎); make the tip point along the running direction of meridian-qi and puncture with inserting manipulation, which is considered as Sui(Following 随)". In short, after arrival of the needling sensation, puncturing with the needle tip pointing to the running direction of the meridian is taken as rein-forcing; on the contrary, puncturing with the tip of the needle against the course of the meridian is taken as reducing. This method is only one of the reinforcing-reducing manipulations by punc-turing along and against the direction of the meridian as related in ancient books.

5. Reinforcing and Reducing by Manipulating the Needle in Cooperation with the Patient's Respiration

Differentiation of reinforcing and reducing is based on whether the needle is inserted during the patient's inspiration and withdrawn during the patient's expiration or vice versa. That is, the differentiation of the two is based on the relationship between the needle insertion and withdrawal and patient's inspiration and expiration.

Plain Questions(素问, Su Wen) says that, "Insert the needle during the patient's inspira-tion, do not exhale the air, ···. withdraw the needle during his expiration and retreat the needle out at the end of the exspiration to make all the evils be removed, which is termed reducing. In-sert the needle at the end of the patient's exspiration, ···. withdraw it during his inspiration, keep vital energy retained in the respective area of the body, ···make the vital energy circulate in the body, which is termed reinforcing. " These two quotations point out that if the needle is inserted when the patient inhales the air and withdrawn when the patient exhales the air, this manipula-tion is taken as reducing; If the needle is inserted when the patient exhales the air and withdrawn when the patient inhales the air, it is taken as reinforcing. *Great Compendium of Acupuncture and Moxibustion*(针灸大成, Zhen Jiu Da Cheng) further states in detail that, "If reinforcing is required to be achieved, insert the needle during the patient's expiration and withdraw it during the patient's inspiration; if the reducing is required to be achieved, insert the needle during the patient's inspiration and withdraw the needle during the patient's expiration". This kind of rein-forcing-reducing manipulation is usually combined with the lifting-thrusting and twisting meth-ods to strengthen the reinforcing or reducing effect.

6. Reinforcing and Reducing by Keeping the Needling Hole Open or Close

Differentiation of reinforcing and reducing is based on whether the hole the needle makes is pressed and closed immediately after the needle is withdrawn.

Miraculous Pivot(灵枢, Ling Shu) says that, "The reducing···, shaking the needle after it is inserted to increase the size of the punctured hole so that Qi disperses easily; the reinforcing ···. , kneading or pressing the punctured hole after the needle is withdrawn and have it closed so that qi is kept inside. " *Plain Questions*(素问, Su Wen) says that, "As far as the reinforcing and reducing by puncturing is concerned, the right hand is used to hold the needle and the left used to press the puncturing hole. For the patient with excess syndrome, the hole is left untouched to al-low outward flow of qi; for the patient with deficiency syndrome, the hole should be pressed and closed to avoid the outward flow of qi. " What these two quotations state is that after the needle is withdrawn, swiftly pressing and closing the punctured hole may retain the genuine qi, which is taken as reinforcing; Shaking the needle to enlarge the size of the puncturing hole without press-ing may leave the pathogenic qi disperse, which is taken as reducing.

The basic reinforcing and reducing manipulations above are summarized up as follows. (See Tab. 2—3)

Tab. 2－3   Basic Reinforcing and Reducing Manipulations

Name	Reinforcing manipulation	Reducing manipulation
Reinforcing and reducing by lifting and thrusting the needle	Thrust the needle from the shallow portion of the acupoint to the deep portion; thrust the needle quickly and heavily and lifting it slowly and gently	Lift the needle from the deep portion of the acupoint to the shallow portion; lifting the needle heavily and quickly and thrust it gently and slowly
Reinforcing and reducing by twirling and rotating the needle	Twist the needle with the thumb moving forward and index finger moving backward (Left turn, i. e. clockwise rotation)	Twist the needle with the thumb moving backward and index finger moving forward (Right turn; i. e. counter-clockwise rotation)
Reinforcing and reducing by rapid and slow insertion and withdrawal of the needle	Insert the needle slowly and withdraw the needle quickly; insert the needle from the shallow portion of the acupoint to the deep portion; three needle insertions and one needle withdrawal	Insert the needle swiftly and withdraw it slowly; withdraw the needle from the deep portion of the acupoint to the shallow portion; one needle insertion and one needle withdrawal
Reinforcing and reducing by puncturing along and against the direction of the meridian	Insert or operate the needle along the direction of the meridian	Insert or operate the needle against the direction of the meridian; weaken qi-circulation along with the manipulation
Reinforcing and reducing by manipulating the needle in cooperation with the patient's respiration	Insert the needle during the patient's expiration and withdraw the needle during the patient's inspiration	Insert the needle during the patient's inspiration and withdraw it during the patient's expiration
Reinforcing and reducing by keeping the needle hole open or closed	Press and close the punctured hole immediately after the needle is withdrawn	Pressing the punctured hole slowly or shake the needle to enlarge the hole

7. Heat-Inducing Needling(Reinforcing Needling)

This is a comprehensive reinforcing method consisting of four basic reinforcing manipulations: manipulations by rapid and slow insertion and withdrawal of the needle, by lifting and thrusting the needle, by nine-six multiples, and by keeping the punctured hole open or close.

The book *Songs of Golden Needles*(金针赋, Jin Zhen Fu) says that, "Heat-inducing puncture treats obstinate numbness and cold-pain. Puncture shallow and then deeply, operate three-insertings and three-drawings nine times, lift the needle slowly and thrust it quickly until a heat sensation is produced, withdraw the needle and press the point to close the hole. It can eliminate cold evil." *Great Compendium of Acupuncture and Moxibustion*(针灸大成, Zhen Jiu Da Cheng) also explains "Heat-inducing puncture can clear away cold···. Three insertions and one drawing ···. insert the needle for 0. 5 cun and twirl it nine times···. Thrust it gradually to 1. 0 cun, operate the manipulations of three-drawings and three-thrustings with slow lifting and quick thrusting.

If there's a tight sensation under the needle, heat-qi will be produced, and cool-qi will be eliminated. If there is no such an effect, repeat the procedure again." In summary, after inserting the needle into the skin and the needling appears, divide the acupoint, based on the depth of it, into the shallow, middle and deep portion, or only the shallow and deep portion. Thrust the needle quickly (forcefully) and lift it slowly (gently) for nine times at the shallow portion. Then insert the needle down to the middle and the deep portion and thrust and lift the needle at the different layers in the same way as at the shallow portion for the same nine times, which is called the first degree. (See Fig. 2—25). After that, withdraw the needle to the shallow portion and repeat this course until the patient complains of hot sensation at the punctured area. Then, withdraw the needle out of the body and quickly press the punctured hole. In this operation, the reinforcing manner by inserting the needle during the patient's expiration and withdrawing it during the patient's inspiration can be applied in coordination.

This heat-producing needling method is to make Yang-qi enter into the interior of the body and a warm sensation to appear at the local area or in the whole body. The theoretical basis of this method lies in the saying that, "Puncturing for defficiency can bring about excess which produces heat around the needling area. Only strong qi can induce heat sensation." which was recorded in *Plain Questions* (素 问, Su Wen). When administering this method, it is advisable to do it at the area where the muscles are abundant and thick. For the patient who is sensitive to acupuncture, the manipulation should not be too violent so as to prevent the patient from fainting. After several courses, if the patient still does not have the warm sensation, this manipulation should be stopped, or some sequelae may appear.

8. Cool-Inducing Needling (Reducing Needling)

This method corresponds with (is opposite to) the heat-producing needling and is a comprehensive reducing method which is made up of the four basic reducing manipulations (manipulations by rapid and slow insertion and withdrwal of the needle, by lifting and thrusting the needle, by nine-six multiple and by keeping the needling hole open or close).

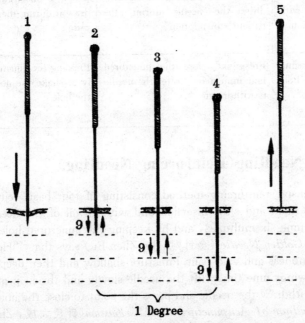

Fig. 2—25   **Heat-Producing Needling**

Songs of Golden Needles(金针赋，Jin Zhen Fu) says that，"Cool-inducing puncture treats the muscular or bone-heat syndrome. Puncture deep and then shallow，operate three-drawings and three-insertings six times；lift the needle quickly and thrust it slowly，then retreat the needle slowly step by step. It can clear away heat evils." *Great Compendium of Acupuncture and Moxibustion*(针灸大成，Zhen Jiu Da Cheng) also says that，"Cool-inducing puncture can clear away heat···. three-drawings and one-inserting with cool sensation···，when needling a point，insert the needle for 1. 0 cun and then twirl it six times···; If getting the needling sensation，lift it for 0. 5 cun，do the manipulation of three-insertions and three-drawings with forceful lifting and gentle thrusting. If there's a tight feeling under the needle，slowly retreat the needle out and the cool-qi can be produced. If the effect is not achieved，do it again as mentioned above. "In short，after inserting the needle into the skin and the needle sensation is attained，divide the acupoint，based on the depth of it，into the shallow，middle and deep portion，or only the shallow and deep portion. Lift the needle quickly(forcefully) and thrust it slowly(gently) for six times at the deep portion，then lift the needle up to the middle and shallow portions，thrust and lift the needle in the same way as at the shallow portion for the same six times，which is called the first degree(See Fig. 2 —26). After that，thrust the needle to the deep portion and repeat this course until the patient has a cool sensation at the needling area. When the needle is being withdrawn，shake the needle body to increase the size of the hole and leave it untouched to allow outward flow of qi. In this operation，the reducing manner by withdrawing the needle during the patient's expiration and inserting the needle during the patient's inspiration can be applied in coordination.

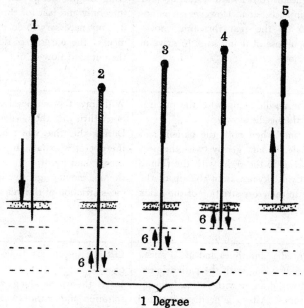

Fig. 2—26   **Cool-Producing Needling**

This cool-producing needling method may make Yin-qi of the body to disperse exteriorly and induce cool sensation in the local area or all over the body.

This method is applicable to heat syndrome due to the attack of pathogenic heat or hyperactivity of Yang-qi.

Contrast between heat-producing and cool-produing needlings, See Tab. 2—4.

Tab. 2－4 **Contrast between Heat-Producing and Cool-Producing Needlings**

Step	Heat-producing needling	Cool-producing needling
1	More expiration and less inspiration, insert the needle with the expiration Ask the patient to inhale air with the nose and exhale air with the mouth; short-time inspiration and long-time expiration (One inspiration and three expirations)	Much inspiration and less expiration, insert the needle along with the inspiration Ask the patient to exhale air with the nose and inhale air with the mouth Long-time inspiration and short-time expiration (three inspirations and one expiration)
2	First shallow, then deeply, twist the needle left along with the patient's expiration. First insert the needle into a certain depth, after there a needling sensation appears, lifting the needle 0. 5 cun up, hold the needle and ask the patient to continue respiration with long expiration and short inspiration. Then, during the patient's expiration, twist the needle left for one turn with the thumb moving forward and the index finger backward. The finger force should be exerted on the thumb. Meanwhile, by way of quivering of the hand, thrust the needle downward forcefully for three times in succession. However, it is not necessary to do the real thrusting movements, the purpose of doing so is to drive qi into the interior	First deeply, then shallowly, twist the needle right along with the patient's inspiration First insert the needle to a certain depth and after a needling sensation occurs, thrust the needle about 1 cun deep, holding the needle and asking the patient to continue the respiration with long inspiration and short expiration. Then, during the patient's inspiration, twist the needle right for one turn with the index finger moving forward and the thumb backward. The finger force should be exerted on the index finger. Meanwhile, by the quivering of the hand, lift the needle upward forcefully and fast for three times. However, it is not necessary to do the real lifting movements, the purpose of doing so is to induce the outward flow of qi
3	Withdraw the needle along with the inspiration, lifting the needle slowly. During the time when both the patient and operator inhale the air, gently twist the needle and return it to the right with the thumb moving gently backward from the tip of the index finger to the cross striation of the index finger	Withdraw the needle along with the expiration, thrusting the needle slowly. During the time when both the patient and the operator exhale the air gently twist the needle and return it to the left with the thumb moving gently backward from the cross striation of the index finger to the tip of this finger
4	Thrust the needle nine times and lift it once. Insert the needle along with the patient's expiration and withdraw it with patient's inspiration nine times. After the needle is inserted gradually into the deep portion of the acupoint, lift it to the original shallow portion; repeat the movements in the same way as the above	Lift the needle six times and thrust it only once Insert the needle along with the patient's inspiration and withdrawing it along with the patient's inspiration for six times. After the needle is withdrawn gradually to the shallow portion of the acupoint, thrust it into the original deep portion. Repeat the movements in the same way as above

Step	Heat-producing needling	Cool-producing needling
5	Concentrate the mind and repeat the operation Always having the needle in the hand. Concentrate the mind and repeat the operation with the respiration of both the patient and the clinician Insert the needle heavily and withdraw the needle gently (inserting the needle quickly for three times and withdrawing the needle slowly only once); Use more left turns (clockwise rotation) with less right turns (counter clockwise rotation). Insert the needle with expiration and withdraw the needle with inspiration until the patient has a hot sensation in the needling area which spreads around along the meridian	Concentrate the mind and repeat the operation Always having the needle in the hand, concentrating the mind and repeating the operation along with the respiration of both the patient and the clinician. Keep in mind that withdrawing the needle heavily and inserting the needle gently (withdrawing the needle quickly ror three times and inserting the needle slowly only once). is necessary More right turn (counter-clockwise rotation) with less left turns (clockwise rotation). Insert the needle with inspiration and withdraw it with expiration until the patient complains of hot sensation at the punctured area which spreads along the meridian
6	Incline the needle body with the tip pointing to the diseased area, inducing the qi to move forward Withdraw the needle 0.5 cun deep, incline the needle shaft with the tip pointing to the diseased part, or to the running direction of the course of the meridian; Shake the needle along with the patient's expiration, withdraw and turn it left forcefully. Then, shake the needle again along with the patient's inspiration and twisting it gently and turn it to the right	Inclin the needle body with the tip pointing to the diseased area, inducing outward flow of qi Withdraw the needle 0.5 cun up, inclining the needle shaft with the tip pointing to the diseased area, or with the tip against the running direction of the course of the meridian, shaking the needle along with the patient's inspiration, lifting and turning it right forcefully; Then, shak the needle again along with the patient'is expiration and twist it gently and turn it to the left
7	Stop operation and regulate qi, scrap the handle downward Holding the needle and insert it perpendicularly, thrusting it again with slight twirling, retaining it in the acupoint. Then, with the index and middle fingers hold the shaft of the needle, scrape the handle downward with the thumb nail for 5 — 7 times every 5 — 7 breaths.	Stop manipulation and regulate qi, scrape the handle upward Hold the needle without inserting it, after twirling the handle slightly and inserting it into the acupoint. Then, with the index and middle finger holding the shaft of the needle, scrape the handle upward with the thumb nail for 5—7 times every 5—7 breaths.
8	Withdraw the needle along with the inspiration and press the needle opening quickly Withdraw the needle out of the body along with the patient's inspiration. When doing so, withdraw the needle directly without shaking it. After withdrawal of the needle, press the punctured hole swiftly	Withdraw the needle along with the expiration without press the needle opening Withdraw the needle out of the body along with the patient's expiration. When doing so, the needle is shaken. After withdrawal of the needle, do not press the punctured hole

In summary, these two kinds of comprehensive reinforcing and reducing methods(i. e. the heat-producing and cool-producing needlings) are, in fact, the combination of several different manipulations to reinforce and reduce. That is, the manipulation by rapid and slow insertion and withdrawal of the needle which is characterized by "three insertions and one withdrawal" or "one insertion and three withdrawals", the manipulation by lifting and thrusting the needle in terms of nine-yang or six-yin numbers which is manifested as quick thrusting and slow lifting, or quick lifting and slow thrusting and the manipulation by keeping the punctured hole open or closed. The so-called "three insertions and one withdrawal" refers to the dividing of the punctured acupoint into shallow(heaven), middle(man) and deep(earth) portions and inserting the needle from the shallow to the middle and then to the deep portion three times and withdrawing it again directly to the shallow portion. It reflects the reinforcing principle of inserting the needle slowly and withdrawing the needle swiftly. The so-called "one insertion and three withdrawal" refers to dividing the punctured acupoint into shallow(heaven), middle(man) and deep(earth) portions. The needle is inserted directly from the shallow portion to the deep portion and then, withdrawn in order from the deep to the middle and then to the shallow portion three times. It reflects the reducing principle of inserting the needle swiftly and withdrawing the needle slowly.

The Chinese character "Jin"(紧) and "Man"(慢) in acupuncture treatment refers to, on the basis of attainment of needling sensation, the heaviness when the force is exerted, and the speed when the operation is done in the manipulation of lifting and thrusting the needle. "Jin (紧)" has the meanings of both "quick and heavy" while "Man(慢)" has the meanings of both "gentle and slow". "Jin(紧)" and "Man(慢)" is the fusion of two opposite movements. In the needling manipulations, they too are represented as "heavy and quick thrusting and gentle and slow lifting "or" heavy and quick lifting and gentle and slow thrusting". (See Fig. 2−23, 2−24)

Moreover, there are other manipulations, such as fire(yang)-producing needling, heat-promoting needling, which are similar to the above heat-producing needling, water(yin)-producing needling and cool-promoting needling, which are similar to the cool-producing needling. (See Tab. 2−5)

9. Yin Occluding in Yang(The Reinforcing Containing the Reducing)

This is a comprehensive needling method for both reinforcing and reducing in combination. It consists of three manipulations: rapid and slow insertion and withdrawal of the needle, thrusting and lifting the needle and the nine-six multiple method.

Songs of Golden Needles(金针赋, Jin Zhen Fu) says that, "The needling method of Yin occluding in Yang is first to induce heat, then cold, which is special for the syndrome of cold followed by heat. Then, insert the needle shallow and then deep and operate the Nine-six multiple manipulations; i. e. Reinforcing before Reducing. "*Great Compendium Acupuncture and Moxibustion*(针灸大成, Zhen Jiu Da Cheng) also says, "During puncturing, first insert the needle for 0. 5 cun and operate the Nine-time manipulation. Then, if there is a slight hot feeling under it, thrust it to 1. 0 cun and operate the Six-time manipulation to get needling sensation. This is the so-called Yin occluding in Yang, which treats the syndrome of cold followed by heat; i. e. Reinforcing before Reducing. "

Therfore, first, divide the depth of the punctured point into the shallow and deep portion. Then, insert the needle to the shallow portion and induce the needling sensation. At this layer, forcefully thrust and gently lift the needle 9 times until the patient complains of the hot sensation at the local area, then, withdraw the needle out of the body with the punctured hole untouched (without pressing the hole). (See Fig. 2−27)

Tab. 2−5   Fire-producing, Heat-promoting, Water-producing and Cool-promoting needlings

Manipulation	Function	Operation	Remarks
Fire-producing needling	Heat-reinforcing	Insert the needle 0. 1 cun deep, asking the patient to breathe out with the mouth. During his or her expiration, lift and thrust the needle in a 0. 1 cun extent for three times. Then, asking the patient to inhale the air with the nose and exhale the air with the mouth for 3 times. shake the needle and a hot sensation will naturally be induced naturally, repeat this course several times after each insertion for 0. 1 cun deep	These two manipulations are the simplified forms of the commonly used heat-producing and cool-producing needlings. They have less stimulations and the heat and cool sensation they induce only occurs at a local area. But they have the same indications as the heat and cool-producing needlings do.
Water-producing needling	Cool-inducing	Insert the needle 0. 1 cun deep. Ask the patient to breathe in with the mouth and during his or her inspiration, thrusting and lift the needle in a 0. 1 cun extent for three times. Then, ask the patient to exhale the air with the nose and inhaling the air with the mouth three times. Shake the needle and a cool sensation will be induced naturally. Repeat this course for several times after each insertion for 0. 1 cun	
Heat-promoting needling	Heat-reinforcing	Press closely on the acupoint with the index finger of the left hand and hold the needle with the right hand. After the needle is inserted and the sensation is obtained, exert more pressure on the left hand and twist and thrustthe needle with the thumb of the right hand moving forward for 5 seconds. Wait for the arrival of a heavy and tight sensation. Then continuously thrust the needle heavily and lift it gently for ten seconds. Twisting the needle again,more the thumb forward for 45 seconds. Make the needling sensation change to hot sensation, withdraw the needle slowly and press the hole quickly.	These two manipulations need the cooperation of both hands. Special attention should be paid to the presence of the needling sensation. The manipulations not only enable the patient to bring about the hot or cool sensation, but also can make the patient's local temperature go up or down
Cool-promoting needling	Cool-inducing	Press closely on the acupoint with the index finger of the left hand and hold the needle with the right hand. After the needle is inserted and the needling sensation is attained, decrease the pressure exerted by the left hand. Twisting and lifting the needle with the thumb of the right hand move backward for 5 seconds. Then, after the heavy and tight sensation appears, lift and thrust the needle for about one minute, continuously thrusting the needle gently and lifting it heavily for ten seconds and making the needling sensation change to a cool sensation. Withdrawing the needle swiftly with the hole untounched	

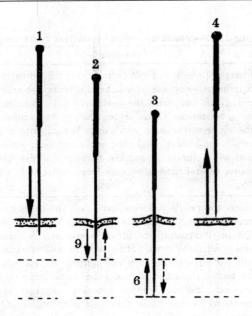

Fig. 2—27 Yin Occluding in Yang

Yang pertains to the reinforcing and Yin to the reducing. The so-called Yin occluding in Yang means that the reinforcing contains the reducing. This method belongs to the one of reinforcing before reducing, which is applicable to syndrome of cold followed by heat, or deficiency complicated with excess.

10. Yang Occluding in Yin(The Reducing Containing the Reinforcing)

Songs of Golden Needles(金针赋，Jin Zhen Fu) says that, "The needling method of Yang occluding in Yin is first to induce cold, then heat, which is special for the syndrome of heat followed by cold. Insert the needle deeply and then shallow and operate the Six-nine multiple manipulations；i. e. Reducing before Reinforcing." *Great Compendium of Acupuncture and Moxibustion*(针灸大成，Zhen Jiu Da Cheng) also says that, "During puncturing, first insert the needle for 1. 0 cun and operate the six-time manipulation. Then, if there's a slight cool feeling under it, withdraw it up to 0. 5 cun. Operate the Nine-time manipulation to get the needling sensation. This is the so-called Yang occluding in Yin, which can treat the syndrome of heat followed by cold；i. e. Reducing before Reinforcing."

The concrete operation is to divide the depth of the punctured point in to the shallow and deep portion. Then, insert the needle to the deep portion and induce the needling sensation there. Then gently thrust and forcefully lift the needle for six times until the patient has a cool sensation. Then, withdraw the needle to the shallow portion and gently lift and forcefully thrust it for nine times. After the patient gains the local sensation, withdraw the needle out of the body and press the hole to close it. (See Fig. 2—28)

Yang pertains to reinforcing and Yin to reducing. Yang occluding in Yin means that the reducing contains reinforcing, it belongs to the method of reducing before reinforcing. This method is suitable for the syndrome of heat followed by cold, or excess complicated by deficiency.

11. Dragon-Tiger Fighting

Great Compendium Acupuncture and Moxibustion(针灸大成，Zhen Jiu Da Cheng) says

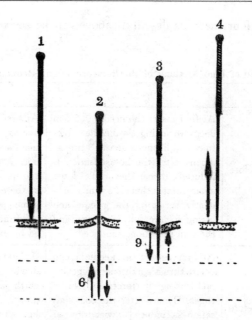

Fig. 2—28 Yang Occluding in Yin

that, "During puncturing, first operate left-dragon manipulation, i. e. twirling the needle left for nine times, which is an odd number. Then, operate the right-tiger manipulation, i. e. twirling the needle right for six times, which is an even number. Operate this method repeatedly with dragon (left) twirling before tiger (right) twirling to reinforce qi after getting the needling sensation. Therefore, the methods of Yin occluding in Yang, Yang occluding in Yin, twirling the needle left for nine times and twirling the needle right for six times can relieve pain. Since this kind of method needs the repeated left and right operations, it is known as "fighting of the Dragon and Tiger" in acupuncture treatment. This is a comprehensive needling method for both reinforcing and reducing in combination, but it emphasizes the manipulation by twirling and rotating the needle and the cooperation of the nine-six multiple method. To its concrete operation, the needle is twirled forcefully clockwise 9 times and twirled again counter clockwise 6 times. This course is repeated several times. If necessary, the twirling of the needle may be conducted at the different shallow, middle and deep portions of the acupoint. "Dragon" here refers to twirling the needle clockwise and "tiger" refers to twirling the needle counter-clockwise. The dragon-tiger fighting refers to the alternation of the clockwise and anti-clockwise twirling manipulation. This method has the functions of regulating Ying and Wei and makes the needling sensation stronger, so it is suitable to induce an analgesic effect.

12. Midnight-Noon Lifting and Thrusting of the Needle

Catechism on Acupuncture and Moxibustion(针灸问对, Zhen Jiu Wen Dui) says that, "After inserting the needle and regulating the respiration, thrust the needle 9 times and then lift it 6 times. At the same time, twist the needle left and right to regulate the Yin-qi and Yang-qi. This method is useful to treat all kinds of diseases. " This is a comprehensive needling manipulation in which the basic thrusting and lifting, the twirling and the nine-six multiple methods are combined. The name "midnight-noon" here refers to the twirling of the needle clockwise and counter-clockwise. To its operation, following the insertion of the needle and after the arrival of needling sensation, the needle is thrusted and twisted clockwise for 9 times and then lifted and twisted anti-clockwise for 6 times. This procedure may be repeated for several times before the needle is withdrawn to conduct Yin-qi and Yang-qi and promote the circulation of the meridian-qi. This mthod is excellent for treating ascites and eructation.

The comparison of the four methods described above can be summarized as follows. (See Tab. 2—6)

Tab. 2—6   Comparison of Four Methods of the Reinforcing and Reducing in Combination

Name	Function	Operation	Remarks
Yin occluding in Yang	Reinforcing before reducing	At first insert the needle 0. 5 cun deep, thrusting the needle forcefully and lifting it gently 9 times. Then, after the hot sensation is induced, thrust the needle down again for another 0. 5 cun deep, gently thrusting the needle and lifting it forcefully 6 times, and the cool sensation is induced.	At first, administer the heat-producing needling method at the main (middle) portion of the acupoint, then, administering the cool-producing needling method at the earth (deep) portion of the same point. Applicable to the syndrome of deficiency complicated by excess.
Yang occluding in Yin	Reducing before reinforcing	At first, insert the needle 1 cun deep, thrusting the needle gently and lifting it forcefully for 6 times. Then, after the cool sensation is induced, withdraw or lift it for 0. 5 cun, forcefully thrusting the needle and gently lifting it for 9 times, and the hot sensation is induced.	At first, conducting the cool-producing needling method at the earth (deep) portion of the acupoint. Then, conducting the heat-produccion needling method at the heaven (shallow) portion of the same acupoint. Applicable to the syndrome of excess complicated with deficiency
Dragon-tiger fighting	Reinforcing before reducing; Removing pathogenic factors and relieving pain	At first, administer the "Green Dragen Shaking Tail" method, twisting the needle clockwise for 9 times, then, administering the "White tiger Shaking Head" method, twisting the needle anticlockwise for 6 times.	Emphasize the manipulation of twisting clockwise for 9 times and counter-clockwise for 6 times
Midnight-noon thrusting and lifting of the needle	Treating ascites and eructation	When inserting the needle, regulat the respiration, thrusting the needle quickly for 9 times and lifting it quickly for 6 times. Meanwhile, twisting the needle clockwise and conntor-clockwise in coordination to conduct Yin-qi and Yang-qi	Emphasize the manipulation of thrusting the needle for 9 times and lifting it for 6 times

Appendix 1   Uniform Reinforcing and Reducing Method and Qi-Inducing Method

The uniform reinforcing and reducing method applied in modern clinic is a kind of needling therapy in which the attainment of needling sensation is the main purpose without administering any special reinforcing-reducing manipulation. Usually this method is conducted by administering a small amplitude lifting-thrusting, or low-frequency twirling manipulation after the needle sensation is obtained. Then, the needle is retained or withdrawn immediately.

This method is suitable for patients with deficiency syndrome or the ones with mild excess syndrome, or those who are particularly insensitive to acupuncture treatment. It is also applicable to chronic cases with both excess and deficiency syndromes.

The so-called uniform reinforcing and reducing method probably originated with the Qi-inducing method recorded in *Miraculous Pivot*(灵枢, Ling Shu) which says that, "Qi-inducing is the slow thrusting and lifting of the needle". After the needling sensation is obtained, slowly and evenly lift, thrust, twist and twirl the needle to recover the meridian-qi to normality. *Miraculous Pivot*(灵枢, Ling Shu) also says that, "The disorders due to excess or deficiency of meridian-qi are the result of the disability of qi-flowing." The qi-inducing method is suitable for the patient whose meridian-qi is not functioning properly but whose visceral-qi is not dysfunctional. This method may conduct and direct the meridian-qi, avoiding the entrance of the pathogenic qi into the interior, thereby attaining the purpose of treating the disease.

Appendix 2   The Strong and Weak Stimulation

It is generally regarded that the reducing puncture is strong stimulation and the reinforcing is weak stimulation. But from the view point of clinical practice, it is not always the case. The reinforcing sometimes includes a strong stimulation while the reducing maybe include a weak one. For instance, though the heat-producing needling is the reinforcing and cool-producing needling is the reducing, they both belong to strong stimulations. So, in the clinic, that the choice of a strong or weak stimulation should be made is based on the principle of "treatment according to the syndrome differentiation" and the practical requirements. Only in this way, can the curative effect be increased.

Appendix 3   The Other Reinforcing and Reducing Methods

They are related as follows. (See Tab. 2—7)

VIII. Manipulations of Retaining and Withdrawing the Needle

1. Retaining the Needle

Retaining the needle refers to the method by which the needle is kept in the acupoint after it is inserted. During the retaining process, the needle can be retained statically in the body, which is known as "static needle retention", or manipulated intermittently to increase the needle sensation and prolong the needling intensity, which is termed as "dynamic needle retention."

In general, so long as the needle sensation has arrived around the needle and the manipulations have been finished, the needle can be withdrawn, or if not, retained for 10—20 minutes according to the different conditions.

Clinically, the determination of needle it and the duration of the retention depend upon, or vary with, different disease, person, season and the location of the acupoint. For example, for chronic, painful and spastic diseases, for patients with a good constitution, for the acupoint where the muscle and skin are thick, or during autumn and winter, the needle-retaining time is often appropriately prolonged. At present, it is generally believed that the needle-retaining method is suitable for reinforcing the deficiency, so this method is often used for deficient syndromes, cold syndromes and chronic diseases.

Retaining the needle is an important link in the whole acupuncture process. If the needle sensation has not arrived, it can aid in its arrival. If the needle sensation has already been induced, it can help remove the pathogen. It can also assist in reinforcing and reducing. If the clinician can properly control the retention of the needle based on the principle of differentiation of the sign and symptoms, he or she can enhance the curative effect further.

Tab. 2—7 The Other Reinforcing and Reducing Methods

Manipulation	Function	Operation	Remarks
Qi-retaining method	Promoting the circulation of qi to dispel accumulation	Insert the needle into the acupoint 0.7 cun deep (human portion, thrusting the needle quickly and lifting it slowly nine times. Then, after presence of the needling sensation, thrust the needle 1 cun deep (earth portion). Slightly lift it 6 times and withdraw it to the original place. If no needling sensation is felt, repeat the procedure until the sensation is obtained.	Treat masses in the hypochondrium or abdomen; Applicable to deficiency-syndrome complicated with excess
Qi-conducting method	Removing pathogenic qi	After inserting the needle into the skin, first administer the needling manipulation 9 times. If the patient has a feeling of fullness at the local area, incline the needle and ask the patient to inhale air for 5 times to conduct the needling sensation to the diseased area.	Treat painful diseases
Qi-lifting method	Reducing before reinforcing	After inserting the needle into the skin, first administer the needle manipulation 6 times. If a needling sensation occurs, slightly twist and gently lift the needle to activate the meridian and its colleterals	Treat numbness due to cold, stubborn arthralgia
Qi-regulating method	Removing accumulation	After inserting the needle into the skin, first administer the Qi-conducting manipulation for 9 or 6 times, then, incline the needle to induce Qi to the diseased area. After the needling sensation arrives, withdraw the needle immediately	

2. Withdrawing the Needle

After manipulating the needle or retaining the needle, the clinician must withdraw the needle. Withdrawing the needle is the last step in the manipulations. When withdrawing the needle, press a dry sterilized cotton ball, which is held with the thumb and index finger of the left hand, around the point. Slowly lift the needle to the subcutaneous part with the right hand after twirling the needle gently, then withdraw the needle. *Great Compendium on Acupuncture and Moxibustion*(针灸大成, Zhen Jiu Da Cheng) says that, "Withdrawing of the needle consists in slowness; Rapid operation usually causes injury." This means that the clinician should withdraw the needle slowly and gently. It is not advisable to pull the needle out rapidly. But for the acupoint which is punctured superficially, rapid withdrawal is better as this method has the advantage of being painless. Attention should be paid to rapid withdrawal of the needle. It should be done evenly and gently.

In addition, withdrawing the needle directly affects the method of reinforcing or reducing by keeping the hole open or closed. That is, do not shake and enlarge the needling hole and close the hole immediately with the cotton ball after the needle is withdrawn so as to keep the genuine qi inside the body to enhance the reinforcing, which is called the reinforcing method. If the needling hole is shaken and enlarged and kept open after the needle is withdrawn to let out the pathogenic qi, this method is called the reducing method.

In order to avoid forgetting the withdrawal of the needles in the body, the clinician should check the number of the needles after finishing the treatment. Also the patient should keep the area around the points clean to avoid the occurrence of infection.

Ⅸ. Point-Penetrating Manipulation

Point penetration method refers to the puncture with a filiform needle from one point to another. Thus, puncturing both points or more with one needle is termed acupoint penetration technique. This technique started in the Jin or Yuan dynasty and it was recorded in the Books of *A Handbook of Prescriptions for Emergency*(肘后备急方, Zhou Hou Bei Ji Fang), *Songs of Jade Dragon*(玉龙歌, Yu Long Ge) and *Compendium of Medicine* (医学纲目, Yi Xue Gang Mu).

This technique is characterized by stimulating more points with less needles. The application of this technique is classified as follows: ① Penetrating points on the same meridian, ② Penetrating points on both the meridians and its adjacant meridian, and ③ Penetrating points on the externally-internally related meridians. According to the angle of needling, the penetration can be classified as the horizontal, oblique and perpendicular. The commonly used acupoints for penetration technique are shown as follows. (See Tab. 2—8)

Tab. 2—8   **The Commonly Used Acupoints for Penetration Technique and Their Clinical Application**

Name of the acupoints	Indications	Manipulations
Baihu(DU20) to Sishencong(EX-HN1)	Headache, dizziness, disorders of eye and nose, prolapse of anus, protracted diarrhea and dysentery, prolapse of uterus, epilepsy, infantile convulsion	Penetrate to Baihui(DU20) subcutaneously along the shin from the points I cun anterior, posterior and lateral to Baihui
Yangbai(GB14) to Yuyao (EX-HN4)	Pain in forehead, trigeminal neuralgia, deviation of the eyes and mouth, redness swelling and pain of the eye.	Insert the needle from Yangbai, penetrate to Yuyao subcutaneously with 1.5 cun needle
Yintang (EX — HN3) to Biliang (Nose Bridge)	Fore-headache, stuffy nose, rhinorrhea	Penetrate from Yintang toward downward subcutaneously I cun alone the midline with 1.5 cun needle.
Sizhukong (SJ 23) to Tongziliao(GB1)	Redness swelling and pain of the eye, lacmination deviation of the eyes and mouth	Penetrate subcutaneously from Sizhukong to Tongziliao with 1.5 cun needle

Name of the acupoints	Indications	Manipulations
Sizhukong（SJ 23） to Shuaigu(GB8)	Migraine, dizziness, infantile convulsion	Penetrate subcutaneously 2-2.5 cun from Sizhukong to Shuaigu with 3 cun needle.
Taiyang （EX-HN5） to Shuaigu(GB 8)	Migraine, dizziness, redness swelling and pain of the eye, infantile corwulsion	Puncture subcutaneously from Taiyang to Shuaigu 2-2.5 cun with 3 cun needle.
Taiyang （EX-HN5） to Quanliao(SI 18)	Toothache, trigeminal neuralgia, deviation of the eye and mouth	Penetrate obliquely 1.5-2 cun from Taiyang, through the medial surface of the zygomatic arch to Quanliao, with 2.5 cun needle
Taiyang （EX-HN 5） to Xiaguan （ST 7）	Toothache, trigeminal neuralgia, deviation of the eye and mouth	Penetrate obliquely 1.5-2 cun from Taiyang, through the medial surface of the zygomatic arch to Xiaguan, with 2.5 cun needle.
Hanyan (GB 4) to Xuanli (GB 6)	Migraine, dizziness, tinnitus	Penetrate subcutaneously from Hanyan to Xuanli 1-1.5 cun with 2 cun needle
Ermen （SJ 21） to Tinghui (GB 2)	Tinnitus, deafness	Open the mouth, penetrate obliquely 1-1.5 cun from Ermen to Tinghui with 2 cun needle.
Dicang (ST 4) to Daying (ST 5)	Toothache, deviation of the eye and mouth, facial spasm	Penetrate subcutaneously 1.5 cun from Dicang to Daying with 2 cun needle
Dicang (ST 4) to Jiache (ST 6)	Deviation of the eye and mouth, facial spasm	Penetrate subcutaneously 2 cun from Dicang to Jiache with 2.5 cun needle
Dicang (ST 4) to Quanliao (SI 18)	Deviation of the eye and mouth, facial spasm, toothache	Penetrate from Dicang to Quanliao with 2.5 cun needle
Dicang (ST 4) to Juliao (ST 3)	Deviation of the eye and mouth, epistaxis, Nasal obstruction	Penetrate subcutaneously 1—1.5 cun from Dicang to Juliao with 2.5 cun needle
Dicang (ST 4) to Yingxiang (LI 20)	Epistaxis, nasal obstruction, deviation of the eye and mouth	Penetrate subcutaneously 1—1.5 cun from Dicang to Yingxiang with 2.5 cun needle
Jiache (ST 6) to Daying (ST 5)	Deviation of the eye and mouth toothache	Penetrate subcutaneously 1—1.5 cun from Jiache to Daying with 2 cun needle
Jiache (ST 6) to Xiaguan (ST 7)	Toothache, deviation of the eye and mouth	Penetrate subcutaneously 1—1.5 cun from Jiache to Xiaguan with 2.5 cun needle

Name of the acupoints	Indications	Manipulations
Tinghui (GB 2) to Yifeng (SJ 17)	Deviation of the eye and mouth, toothache, tinnitus, deafness	Open the mouth, penetrate obliquely 1—1.5 cun from Tinghui to Yifeng with 2 cun needle
Sibai (ST 2) to Yingxiang (LI 20)	Biliary oscariosis, toothache, deviation of the eye and mouth	Penetrate subcutaneously 1—1.5 cun from Sibai to Yingxiang with 2 cun needle
Fengchi (GB 20) to Fengchi (GB 20)	Common cold, pain in the back of the head	Penetrate 1-1.5 cun from the right Fengchi point to the other one with 2.5 cun needle
Tiantu (RN 22) to Huagai (RN 20)	Dysphagia, cough, asthma, pain in the chest	Penetrate from Tiantu to Huagai 2 cun along the posterior aspect of the sternum
Danzhong (RN 17) to Xuanji (RN 21)	Cough, asthma, pain in the chest	Penetrate subcutaneously 2 cun from Danzhong to Xuanji with 3 cun needle
Danzhong (RN 17) to Zhongting (RN 16)	Dysphagia, cough, asthma, pain in the chest	Penetrate subcutaneously 1 cun from Denzhong to Zhongting with 2 cun needle
Danzhong (RN 17) to Ruzhong (ST 17)	Acute mastitis, scant breast milk	Penetrate subcutaneously 1-1.5 cun from Danzhong to Ruzhong with 2 cun needle
Chengman (ST 20) to Liangmen (ST 21)	Biliary ascariasis, pain in epigastrium and abdomen	Penetrate obliquely 1 cun from Chengman to Liangmen with 1.5 cun needle
Huaroumen (ST 24) to Liangmen (ST 21)	Gastroptosis, epigastralgia	Penetrate obliquely 2 cun from Huaroumen to Liangmen with 3 cun needle
Guanyuan (RN 4) to Qugu (RN 2)	Anuresis, enuresis, seminal emission, impotence, Ieukorrhea, irregular menstruation, amenorrhea, pralapse of uterus	Penetrate obliquely 2 cun from Guanyuan to Qugu with 3 cun needle
Xinshu (BL 15) to Shendao (DU 11)	Angina pectoris, palpitation, cardiolgia, acute mastitis	Penetrate 1.5 cun from Xinshu to Shendao with 2 cun needle, form an angle of 40° with the skin surface
Yaoqi (EX — B9) to Yaoyangguan (DU 3)	Epilepsy, acute lumber sprain, pain in the lower limb	Prone posture, penetrate 1-1.5 cun subcutaneously from the sacral hiatus to Yaoyang guan along the region between the sacrum and skin, with 3 cun needle

Name of the acupoints	Indications	Manipulations
Changqiang (DU 1) to Yaoshu (DU 2)	Prolapse of the rectum, epilepsy	Penetrate 2.5 cun subcutaneously from Changqiang to Yaoshu with 3 cun needle
Hegu (LI 4) to Laogong (PC 8)	Dysphagia, toothache, pain in shoulder and arm	Penetrate 1-1.2 cun from Hegu to Laogong along the palmar with 1.5 cun needle
Hegu (LI 4) to Houxi (SI 3)	Acute lumbar sprain, pain in shoulder and back, numbness of the fingers, convulsion	Penetrate 2.5 cun perpendicularly from Hegu to Huoxi along the palmar of the metacarpal bone, with 3 cun needle
Sanjian (LI 3) to Hegu (LI 4)	Constipation, accumulation of fluid due to febrile disease	Penetrate obliquely 1.2 cun from Sanjian to Hegu with 2 cun needle
Neiguan (PC 6) to Waiguan (SJ 5)	Contusion in the chest and back, asthma, malaria	Penetrate perpendicularly 1.5 cun from Neiguan to Waiguan with 2 cun needle
Neiguan (PC 6) to Ximen (PC 4)	Angina pectoris, palpitation, vomiting, stomachache	Penetrate obliquely 2 cun from Neiguan to Ximen, with 3 cun needle from an angle of 30° with the skin surface
Jianshi (PC 5) to Zhigou (SJ 6)	Malaria, asthma, pain in the chest and back or hypochondriac region	Penetrate perpendicularly 1.5 cun from Jianshi to Zhigou with 2 cun needle
Quchi (LI 11) to Shaohai (HT 3)	Hypertension, pain in the elbow	Penetrate perpendicularly 2 cun from Quchi to Shaohai with 2 cun needle
Taichong (LR 3) to Yongquan (KI 1)	Hypertension, headache, dizziness, numbness of the toes	Penetrate perpendicularly 2 cun from Taichong to Yongquan with 2 cun needle
Qiuxu (GB 40) to Zhaohai (KI 6)	Coronary heart disease, angina pectoris, pain in the chest, acute mastitis, scant breast milk, pain in the hypochondriac region, monic-depressive psychosis, ankle injury	Insert needle from Qiuxu, penetrate out of Zhaohai with 4 cun needle
Kunlun (BL 60) to Taixi (KI 3)	Pain in the back and loins, stiffneck, flaccidity of the lower limbs, numbness of the foot, dizziness, tinnitus	Insert needle from Kunlun, penetrate out of Taixi with 1.5 cun needle
Xuanzhong (GB 39) to Sanyinjiao (SP 6)	Pain in the shoulder, back and hypochondrial region, stiffneck, pain and numbness in the lower limbs, irregular menstruation, leukorrhea with reddish discharge	Penetrate perpendicularly 2 cun from Xuanzhong to Sanyinjiao with 2.5 cun needle

Name of the acupoints	Indications	Manipulations
Tiaokou (ST 38) to Chengshan (BL 57)	Frozen shoulder, shoulder injury, flaccidity of the lower limbs numbness of the foot	Penetrate perpendicularly 2 cun from Tiaokou to Chengshan with 3.5 cun needle
Yanglingquan (GB 34) to Yinlingquan (SP 9)	Pain in the hypochondrial region, pain in the shoulder or knee arthralgia of lower extremities	Penetrate perpendicularly 3 cun from Yangling quan to Yinling quan with 4 cun needle
Ququan (LR 8) to Xiyangguan (GB 33)	Pain of the knee	Sit up straight, hang the feet and flex the knees in an angle of 90°, penetrate obliquely 2-2.5 cun from Ququan to Xiyangguan with 3 cun needle

Chapter Three

Other Needle Instruments and Their Manipulations in Acupuncture Therapy

Ⅰ. Acupuncture with the Three-Edged Needle

The three-edged needle was also called the ensiform needle in ancient times. The book *Miraculous Pivot*（灵枢，Ling Shu）says, "The disease caused by the obstinate stagnation of qi and blood in the channel system…, and the disease remaining long in the five Zang organs are treated with the ensiform needle. " This book also says, "The needle is tube-shaped, with a triangular head of three sharp edges for treating diseases. It can also be used to purge away heat by blood-letting to cure the obstinate diseases. " This is the earliest account of the use of the three-edged needle to treat diseases. The three-edged needle is commonly used in blood-letting therapy to prick a certain acupoint or superficial blood vessels in the body of a patient to cause bleeding, so as to cure some diseases. This method of needling was also referred to as "meridian and vessel pricking(puncture)" during ancient times. It is now called "blood-letting therapy. "

Chinese forefathers paid particular attention to blood-letting therapy. The *Miraculous Pivot* （灵枢，Ling Shu）states, "To eliminate stagnation in the meridian and vessel, we should let out blood with blood-letting puncture. " The specific methods of blood-letting puncture such as "collateral puncture," "repeated shallow puncture" and "leopard-spot puncture" were also given a full account in the book *Miraculous Pivot*（灵枢，Ling Shu）. It gives a further description on the range of blood-letting puncture. For instance, when apparent blood stasis occurs, with the channel and vessel becoming full, hard, red, and as fine as a needle, or as thick as a chopstick, the best method to cure with no side effects is to employ blood-letting. It is also pointed out in the

Miraculous Pivot(灵枢, Ling Shu) that when relieving a stabbing pain with blood-letting puncture, first ask the patient where the pain started, then puncture it to draw out a little blood. If the pain starts in the head and it is serious, puncture the head first, then the part between the two eyebrows to cause bleeding. If the pain starts in the hands and arms, first puncture the Hand-Shaoyin and Yangming meridians located between the ten fingers of the two hands to cause bleeding. If the aching pain started in the feet and legs, puncture the Foot Yangming meridian between the ten toes to draw a little blood. Furthermore, the *Miraculous Pivot*(灵枢, Ling Shu) deals with the function of the three-edged needle and the different acupoints to be punctured for treating different kinds of diseases by blood-letting puncture. For example, to relieve a sudden pain in the heart, puncture both the Foot Taiyin and Jueyin meridians at the same time to let out a little blood.

1. The Needle Apparatus

The three-edged needle is the derivative of the ancient ensiform needle. The ensiform needle is a type of sharp needle which is ensiform and three-edged in shape used for treating obstinate diseases, according to the *Miraculous Pivot*(灵枢, Ling Shu). The book also says, "The fourth type of needle is the ensiform needle with a tube-shaped body, with a sharp tip and a total length of 1. 6 cun, which is made in the same way as a regular needle." This is the specific description of the ensiform needle used in ancient times. The modern tri-ensiform needle is usually made of stainless steel, a total length of 6cm, a thicker cylindrical handle, a three-edged body and a very sharp tip. (See Fig. 3—1)

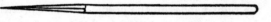

Fig. 3—1 The Three-Edged Needle

2. Manipulation and Procedure

Hold the handle of the needle with the thumb and index finger of the right hand. Support the front part of the needle with the middle finger of the right hand with the tip jutting out slightly to control the depth of the needle. (See Fig. 3—2)
When needling, pinch the area to be punctured with the thumb and index finger of the left hand to make the surface of the skin tight. Then insert the ensiform needle with the right hand into the area.

(1) Spot-Pricking Method.

First press the area above and below the acupoint to be punctured with the thumb and the index finger of the left hand and then move the fingers towards each other to collect the blood in the point to be punctured. Sterilize the skin to be punctured with a cotton ball soaked in 2% tincture of iodine. Then wipe away the iodine with a cotton ball soaked in 75% alcohol. When needling, pinch the position to be punctured tightly with the thumb, index and middle fingers of the left hand. Hold the handle of three-edged needle with the thumb and index finger of the right hand tightly while supporting the lower part of the needle with the middle finger, leaving the tip of the needle exposed. Insert the needle into the sterilized area perpendicularly 0. 1—0. 2 cun. Then withdraw the needle instantly. Slightly squeeze the periphery of the needle hole with the left hand until a little blood flows out. Then cover the hole with a sterilized cotton ball and press slightly. (See Fig. 3—3) This technique is usually applicable for puncturing the tips of the fingers and toes such as the ten Shixuan(EX-UE 11) points and twelve Jing points.

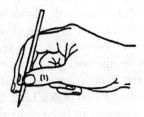

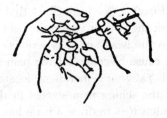

**Fig. 3—2 The Method of Holding
the Three-Edged Needle**

Fig. 3—3   Spot Pricking Method

(2) Scattering Pricking Method

Scattering pricking, also called "leopard-spot needling" during ancient times, means pricking on the periphery of the local affected area. First sterilize the affected area and the acupoint to be punctured. Then prick from the boundary of the affected area to its center. The amount of the pricking depends mainly upon the size of the affected area. (See Fig. 3—4) This kind of needling can remove the local blood stasis and edema, eliminating blood stasis and promoting the circulation of blood as well as possibly clearing and activating the channels and collaterals. This method is usually used to treat local blood stasis, hematoma, edema and chronic eczema.

(3) Blood-Letting Method

First, use the tourniquet to ligate the region proximal to the center to be punctured. Then sterilize the area. Next, press the region inferior to the location to be punctured with the left thumb, hold the needle in the right hand, aim the needle at the vein in the part to be punctured, insert the needle into the vein about 0. 05 — 0. 1 cun; then withdraw it instantly and a small amount of blood will come out. When the blood turns from dark red to bright red, untie the tourniquet. If the blood continues to come out, use a cotton ball to press the needled point to stop bleeding (See Fig. 3—5). The blood-letting method is mainly used at the acupoints of Quze (PC 3) and Weizhong (BL 40) to treat acute vomiting and fever caused by summer-heat evil. The blood-letting therapy is usually conducted once every two or three days. If a patient tends to bleed more than others, the needling can be carried on once every other week or every two weeks. (See Fig. 3—4, 3—5)

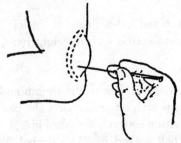

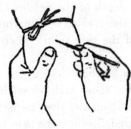

Fig. 3—4   Scattering Pricking Method

Fig. 3—5   Blood-letting Method

(4) Fibre-Tissue-Broken Pricking Method

This is one of the pricking therapies with the three-edged needle. Press two sides of the part to be pricked with the left hand or press from two sides to fix the skin. Hold the needle in the right hand to prick the ster ilized acupoint until some blood or a sticky substance comes out. Or on the basis of the above treatment, prick about 0. 5cm deeper, then tilt the body of the needle to make the tip of the needle more superficial. Then prick out some fiber-like substances from the subcutaneous tissue. Sterilize the pricked part and cover it with an antiseptic.

This method is mainly used at the Back Shu Points which include Xinshu (BL 15), Jueyin

(BL 14),Feishu(BL 13),Ganshu(BL 18),Pishu(BL 20), Shenshu(BL 23),Danshu(BL 19), Weishu(BL 21), Pangguangshu(BL 28), Sanjiaoshu(BL 22),Dachangshu(BL 25),Xiaochangshu(BL 27) and Jiaji(Ex—B2) acupoints. It is also used at painful and reactive points(sensitive spots) and the acupoints distributed on the spinal nervous segments. It is often used to treat diseases like vascular headache, periarthritis of the shoulder,insomnia,cardiac pain,cervical spondylotic syndrome and bronchial asthma.

This fiber-tissue-broken pricking is usually performed once every 3—5 days,3—5 times constituting one course. A second course of treatment starts 10—14 days later.

3. Indications

The three-edged needle is used in blood-letting puncture,so all the diseases caused by stagnation in the meridians and blood stasis, as well as the excess syndrome caused by either inhibitory flow of Yin qi and Yang qi or excessive pathogen, can be treated by applying this kind of needle. All kinds of acupuncture administered with the three-edged needle are aimed at promoting blood circulation, removing swelling, clearing and activating the meridinas and collaterals, and inducing resuscitation by expelling the pathogenic heat. The commonly-used acupoints which deal with three-edged needles are shown in the following. (See Tab. 3—1)

Tab. 3—1 Acupoints and Indications of Blood-letting Puncture with Three-edged Needle

Points	Distribution of blood vessels	Method	Indications
Shixuan (EX-UE 11)	Digital arterial and venous network at each side of the fingers and palm and at the end of the fingers	Blood-letting by pricking method	Fever, coma, heatstroke, syncope, numbness of extremities
Shierjing (Hand)	Digital arterial and venous network at the back of the finger nails and each side of the palm	Blood-letting by pricking method	Fever, coma, sorethroat tonsillitis
Sifeng (EX-UE 10)	Digital arterial and venous network at each side of the palm	Yellow-white liquid being purposely squeezed out after pricking	Infantile malnutrition, whooping, cough, indigestion
Yuji (LU 10)	Venous return branches in thumb	Blood-letting by pricking method and scattered needling	Fever, sore-throat, tonsillitis
Chize (LU 5)	Cephalic vein	Blood-letting by pricking method	Heatstroke, acute vomiting and diarrhen
Quze (PC 3)	Cephalic vein	Blood-letting by pricking method	Heatstroke, stuffiness in chest, vexation
Weizhong (BL. 40)	Great saphenous vein at medial popliteal fossa, small saphenous vein at lateral popliteal fossa	Blood-letting by pricking method	Heatstroke, acute vomiting and diarrhea, systremma

Points	Distribution of blood vessels	Method	Indications
Bafeng (EX-LE 10)	Venous network at the dorsum of the feet	Blood-letting by pricking method	Swelling pain and numbness of foot, bite of a snake in the foot
Baxie (EX-UE 9)	Dorsal venous network of hand	Blood-letting by pricking method	Swelling pain and numbness of hand, bite a of snake in hand
Yintang (EX-HN3)	The branches of artery and vein in medial forehead	Blood-letting by pricking method	Headache, dizziness, conjunctival congestion, rhinitis
Taiyang (EX-HN3)	Venous plexies in fascia	Blood-letting by pricking method and scattered needling	Headache, conjunctival congestion
Baihui (Du 20)	Anastomotic network between the left-right superficial temporal artery and vein and the left-right occipital artery and vein	Blood-letting by pricking method	Headache, vertigo, coma, hypertension
Points at the apex of nose, tragal pit, and ear back	Artery and vein at ear back	Blood-letting by pricking method	Fever, tonsillitis, conjunctival congestion, hypertension
Jinjin, Yuye (EX-HN 13)	Vein of tongue	Blood-letting by pricking method	Wind-stroke syndrome, stiff tongue

4. Precautions

(1) Care must be taken to sterilize properly to prevent infections.

(2) When spot-pricking and scattering pricking are conducted, the manipulation must be gentle, soft, shallow and quick. Be careful not to let out too much blood and never injure the deep big artery when the blood-letting method is used.

(3) In cases of deficiency syndrome, postpartum, spontaneous hemorrhage and haemophilias, this kind of three-edged needle puncture can't be used.

Ⅱ. Acupuncture with the Cutaneous Needle

This cutaneous needle therapy was developed from the therapies of "skin needling", "centro-square needling" and "shallow needling" recorded in *Miraculous Pivot*(灵枢, Ling Shu). This needling method invoives lightly taping certain areas of the skin with short needles and, by means of the actions of the twelve closely-related skin areas and their corresponding acupoints, clear and activate the meridians and collaterals and regulate qi and blood to treat diseases.

1. **Needle Apparatuses and Preparation before Operation**

The head of the cutaneous needle is like a small hammer with a 15—19 cm shaft and a lotus shaped disc attached to one end. Some short small stainless steel needles are embedded under the disc and the number of the embedded needles varies. Based on the shape and number of the needle, they are respectively called plum-blossom needle(five needles), seven-star needle(seven needles) and Luohan needle(eighteen needles). The tips of the needles are not very sharp and should assume a pine-needle-like form. The shaft of needle should be firm and flexible. The tips of all the needles on the disc should be flat and on the same level without any slant, hook, bend, rust, erosion or damage. (See Fig. 3—6).

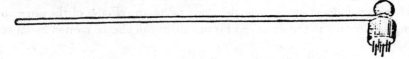

Fig. 3—6   The Cutaneous Needle

Before needling, the needle can be examined by touching the needle tips slightly with a dry and absorbent cotton ball to see whether the needle is hooked or damaged. If the tips become hooked or damaged, cotton fibres will be pulled out easily. Before needling, sterilize the head of the cutaneous needle in 75% alcohol for 30 minutes.

2. **Manipulation and Procedure**

The way of holding the needle is with the right thumb, middle, ring and little fingers. Hold the needle with the end of the handle fixed on the hypothenar eminence of the palm and the middle part of the needle pressed against the extended index finger. (See Fig. 3—7).

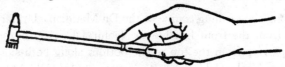

Fig. 3—7   The Method of Holding the Cutaneous Needle

When the cutaneous needle is used to tap around an acupoint on the skin, the head of the needle should be aimed at the skin to be tapped. Using the light, springy force or the flexible movement of the wrist, insert the tips of the needles into the skin and spring them up instantly, like a chicken pecking at the rice. Repeat the tapping again and again. The head of the needle should be perpendicular to the part of the skin. The tapping should be accurate, the speed even and the force used proper. No oblique or slipping puncture is allowed; otherwise, the patient will suffer pain. The interval space or the distance between the tapping spots is usually 1.0—1.5cm.

The tapping manipulation depends on the pathological condition, the location of the disease, the patients' physical constitution and age, and is generally classified as light, heavy and medium. Slight tapping is applied with less force. The shorter the time of contact of the needles with the skin, the better. It is appropriate if the skin becomes slightly red and engorged with blood, without bleeding. Heavy tapping is applied with more force. The time of contact of the tips with the skin is a bit longer. It is appropriate if the skin appears a little bloody. The applied force in medium tapping is between the slight and the heavy. Though this kind of tapping will result in engorged skin red on the tapped part, no blood comes out.

Routine sterilization must be done on the tapped part of the skin.

3. Location of the Tapping

The location of needling with the cutaneous needle is usually classified into three types: tapping along the meridians, on the acupoints and on the affected parts.

1) Tapping along the Meridian Course

This is one of the tapping methods usually used along the Du Meridian and Urinary Bladder Meridian which run through the neck, back and the lumbosacral portion since the Du Meridian can regulate Yang qi of the whole body and all the Back shu points of five zang-organs and six fu-organs distributed on the dorsolumbar region of the Urinary Bladder Meridian. This method is widely used in treating various diseases. Since the source, collateral, vessels, cleft and five Shu points of the twelve meridians spread over the areas below the elbows of the arms and the knees of the legs, diseases related to the Zang and Fu meridians can also be treated by tapping these areas.

2) Tapping the Corresponding Acupoints

The method of tapping on acupoints is based on the principle that where there is an acupoint, there is a cure for disease. The acupoints commonly used in the clinic are the various specific ones such as Huatuojiaji and Ah-shi points.

3) Tapping the Affected Areas

This method is used to tap directly on the area where there is a swelling pain and numbness.
The three tapping methods mentioned above can be used separately or in combination.
The tapping method should be operated in proper order according to the location to be tapped.

(1) Head: Tap along the running course of the Du Meridian, Urinary Bladder Meridian and Gall Bladder Meridian, from the front hairline to Naohu(DU 17), Yuzhen(BL 9) and Fengchi (GB 20). For the temple, tap from the top to the bottom along both sides of the temple.

(2) Nape: Tap from Naohu(DU 17) to the upper Dazhui(DU 14); tap from Fengchi(GB 20), Tianzhu(BL 10) to both sides of Chonggu(EX—HN) at the sixth cervical vertebrae.

(3) Neck:

A) Tap the posterior border of the sternocleidomastoid muscle.

B) Tap downward from the anterior border of the sternocleidomastoid muscle.

C) Tap forward from the posterior angle of the mandible.

(4) Shoulder:

First, tap from top to bottom at the inner fringe of the scapulae; then, tap from inward to outward at the upper fringe of the spina scapulae; finally, tap from inward to outward at the lower fringe of the spina scapulae. Tap heavily around the shoulder joint in the upper front and back axillary fossa if it is difficult for the patient to raise the arms.

(5) Back:

A) Tap the first lateral line of the Urinary Bladder Meridian along both sides of the spinal column.

B) Tap the second lateral line of the Urinary Bladder Meridian along both sides of the spinal column.

(6) Sacral Bone: Tap outward and upward from the tip of coccyx, three parallel lines bilaterally.

(7) Four limbs: Tap along the running course of the three Yang and three Yin Meridians of the hand, the three Yang and three Yin Meridians of the foot; as well as tap around the joints in

a circle.

(8) Face: Tap locally.

(9) Eye:

A) Tap along the eyebrow from the head of the brow to the tail.

B) Tap along the lower border of the orbitae from the inner canthus to Tongziliao(GB 1)

(10) Nose: Mainly tap the cartilages on both sides of the alae of the nose.

(11) Ear: Mainly tap the back of the ear lobes and the external pinna of the ears.

4. Indications

In the clinic, puncture with this kind of needle has produced excellent results for many diseases. The following gives an introduction about the common indications and the location for needling and tapping.

Headache: Tap the occiput, nape and the distal and proximal sensitive regions of the running course of the corresponding meridians.

Migraine: Tap the occiput, nape and the proximal sensitive region of the running course of the corresponding meridians.

Chest pain: Tap along both sides of the thoracic vertabrae (from the first to the twelfth), especially the area of Geshu(BL 17) and Ganshu (BL 18). The tapping can be done up and down along the rib of the painful region.

Pain in hypochondrium: Do the tapping in the same way as done with chest pain. In addition, tap the acupoints of Zhigou(SJ 6) and Taichong(LR 3).

Insomnia: Tap both sides of the spinal column, the acupoints of Xinshu(BL 15), Ganshu (BL 18) as well as the Heart Meridian of Hand-Shaoyin and the Pericardium Meridian of Hand-Jueyin. For dream-disturbed sleep and palpitations, tap the acupoints of Fengchi(GB 20), Sanyinjiao(SP 6) and the sensitive regions around them.

Pain in limbs: Tap the sensitive points in the Du Meridian, the local painful regions and both sides of the thoracic vertebrae for pain in the upper limbs. Tap the painful region and both sides of the lumbar vertebrae for pain in the lower limbs.

Lumbar sprain: Tap the lumbar, sacral regions or both sides of the lumbar and sacral regions, as well as the sensitive regions in the lower limb part of the Urinary Bladder Meridian.

Facial paralysis: Tap the local parts of the face such as Cuanzhu(BL 2), Tongzilao(BL 1), Dicang(ST 4), Jiache(ST 6), and the distal acupoint of Hegu(LI 4) or the sensitive points in the Large Intestine Meridian of Hand Yangming.

Arthralgia syndrome: Tap both sides of the thoracic vertebrae and joints of shoulder and elbow for pain in upper limbs. Tap both sides of lumbar vertebrae and the painful region for pain in the lower limbs. The parts of the affected region can be violently tapped for blood-letting if there is an arthralgia of heat type with redness and swelling. If the athralgia with local swelling and hydrops occurs, blood-letting can be performed by pricking with a three-edged needle and cupping.

Hiccups: Tap both sides of the thoracic vertebrae(from the ninth to the twelfth), the median line of the abdomen and adjunct acupoints Geshu (BL 17), Ganshu(BL 18), Weishu(BL 21), Tianshu(ST 25) and Daheng(SP 15).

Flaccidity syndrome: Tap both sides of the thoracic vertebrae(from the first to the seventh) and adjunct acupoints of the three Yin and three Yang meridians of the hand for flaccidity present in the upper limbs. Tap both sides of the lumbar vertebrae and sacral vertebrae, and also tap along the three Yin and three Yang meridians of the foot for the flaccidity occurring in the lower limbs. For joint deformity, tap violently around the effected region.

Stomachache: Tap Ganshu(BL 18), Pishu(BL 20), Weishu(BL 21), Zhongwan(RN 12) and the adjunct acupoints Gongsun(SP 4) and Zusanli(ST 36).

Vomiting: Tap Ganshu(BL 18), Pishu(BL 20), Weishu(BL 21), Zhongwan (RN 12), and the adjunct acupoint Neiguan(PC 6).

Abdominal pain: For pain in the upper abdomen, mainly tap both sides of the thoracic vertebrae(from the sixth to the twelfth) and the adjunct acupoints Shangwan(RN 13),Zhongwan (RN 12) and Youmen(KI 21). For pain in the lower abdomen,mainly tap both sides of the lumbar vertebrae(from the first to the fifth) and the adjunct acupoints Guanyuan(RN 4) and Qihai (RN 6).

Asthma: Tap both sides of the thoracic vertebrae, acupoints of Feishu(BL 13),Tanzhong (RN 17) and the adjunct acupoints of Tiantu (RN 22) and Tianshu(ST 25).

Cough: Tap both sides of the thoracic vertebrae, acupoints of Feishu(BL 13),Tanzhong (RN 17)and the adjunct acupoint of Chize(LU 5). For abundant expectoration, acupoint Fenglong(ST 40) is added.

Enuresis: Tap both sides of the lumbar and sacral vertebrae. For adults, add the adjunct acupoints of Qihai(RN 6),Guanyuan(RN 4), and Dahe(KI 12). For infants, Sanyinjiao(SP 6) should be added.

Seminal emission: Tap both sides of lumbar and sacral vertebrae and the median line of the abdomen. In addition,acupoints Ciliao (BL 32) is added. Also Sanyinjiao(SP 6) can be added for poor sleep.

Sexual impotence: Tap both sides of lumbar and sacral vertebrae and the median line of abdomen. In addition,acupoint Ciliao(BL 32) and Dahe(KI 12) are added. Also Sanyinjiao(SP 6) can be added for poor sleep.

Dizziness: Tap the head, the acupoints of Ganshu(BL 18), Shenshu(BL 23) and the adjunct acupoint of Taiyang(EX-HN 5). Also,tap the running course of the Gall Bladder Meridian along the sides of head.

Palpitation: Tap the acupoints of Xinshu(BL 15),Ganshu(BL 18) and the adjunct acupoints of Shenmen(HT 7),Sanyinjiao(SP 6) and Taixi(KI 3).

Dysmenorrhea: Tap both sides of lumbosacral trunk and the parts along the running course of the Ren Meridian and the Kidney Meridian. Mainly tap acupoints Qihai (RN 6), Guanyuan (RN 4) and the adjunct acupoints of Ganshu(BL 18)and Sanyinjiao(SP 6).

Infantile convulsion: Tap acupoints Shixuan(EX 30),Fengchi(GB 20), Dazhui(DU 14) and Shenzhu(DU 12).

Eye diseases: Tap around the eyes and the acupoints of Ganshu(BL 18) Danshu(BL 19) and Shenshu(BL 23). For glaucoma, add the adjunct acupoints Fengchi(GB 20)and Cuanzhu (BL 2). For cataract, add Fengchi(GB 20) and Tongziliao(GB 1). For conjunctivitis, add Taiyang(EX—HN 5), Tongziliao(GB 1) and Cuanzhu(BL 2).

Nasal diseases: Tap the acupoints of Feishu(BL 13),Fengchi(GB 20), Yingxiang(LI 20) and Biyuan(EX) and the adjunct acupoints of Hegu(LI 4) and Yuji(LU 10).

Scrofula: Tap both sides of the thoracic vertebrae(from the fifth to tenth) and also tap the area heavily around the scrofula.

5. Precautions

(1) Before needling,the needle apparatuses should be checked carefully. The tips of the needle should be level without any defects. The handle and the head of the needle should be fixed firmly together.

(2) While tapping,the tips of the needle must be perpendicular to the skin. Do not tap obliquely and slipperily so as to reduce pain.

(3) While tapping along meridians, the interval space or the distance between the two tappings is usually about 1cm and 8—16 times constitute a treatment session.

(4) During tapping,if some blood comes out,the local part of the skin should be cleaned and sterilized in order to prevent infection. If there is an ulcer or injury on the local skin, tapping

should be avoided.

Ⅲ. Acupuncture with the Intradermal Needle

The needling method of the intradermal needle is also called "Embedding Therapy", which developed from the practice of retaining an inserted needle for a certain period of time to maintain or prolong the therapeutic effect. There is a saying in the book *Plain Questions*（素问，Su Wen）that, "The longer the inserted needle is retained, the better the therapeutic effect is. "

1. Needle Apparatuses

There are two types of intradermal needles, the granular(wheat-grain shaped)and the thumb-tack(thumb-pin-shaped). (See Fig. 3—8) The acupuncture therapy with the intradermal needle is to insert the needle into the skin and keep it embedded for a certain period of time to prolong the intradermal stimulation of the points so as to regulate the functions of the meridians and collateral of the Zang and Fu organs.

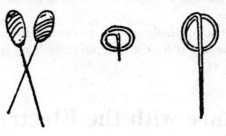

Fig. 3—8　The Intradermal Needle

2. Manipulation and Procedure

First properly sterilize the needles and other instruments to be used, and then the parts of the skin to be needled.

Since the intradermal needle is rather small, and its shape is varied, the method of insertion is different.

(1) Manipulation with the Granular(Wheat-Granule-Shaped) Intradermal Needle

Grip the needle shaft with a pair of tweezers and insert the needle horizontally under the skin at the acupoints. The body of the needle can be embedded for about 3—5 minutes. Then stick a piece of adhesive plaster firmly along the direction of the insertion of the needle. This kind of needle and its needling method are usually used on acupoints on the head, face and back.

(2) Manipulation with the Thumb-tack(Thumb-Pin-Shaped) Intradermal Needle

Grip the ring of the needle with a pair of tweezers and aim the needle tip at the Shu point. Then insert the needle perpendicularly into the skin, embed it and fix it firmly with a piece of adhesive plaster. Or stick the needle ring on a piece of adhesive plaster and apply the plaster together with the needle, perpendicularly to the area to be needled. This kind of needle and its needling manipulation are usually used on the points in the ear.

The duration for retaining the needle depends upon the patient's illness and season of the year. In summer, the needle is usually retained for one or two days and in winter for three to seven days. During the period of embedding, press the embedded needle for one or two minutes every four hours in order to strengthen the stimulation and curative effect.

3. **Indications**

The intradermal needle is commonly used in treating chronic and persistant diseases as well as frequent painful attacks of illness such as nervous headache, stomachache, colicky pain of the gallbladder, asthma, hypertension, neurosism, irregular menstruation, facial spasm and arthralgia syndrome.

4. **Precautions**

(1) Each time, only one or two acupoints are selected which are usually on one side or are the symmetrical ones on both sides.

(2) The needle-embedding therapy is used in parts where the needle can be kept, fixed, and does not hinder the activities of the four limbs. For instance, the needle cannot be embedded in the joints.

(3) After the needle has been embedded, if the patient feels pain or the embedded needle hinders the movement of the limbs, remove it at once and try it again, or select another acupoint.

(4) Before needling, the body of the needle should be checked carefully in order to avoid any accidents.

(5) Pay special attention to cleanliness and sterilization of the needle and puncturing area. In summer, in order to avoid infection, the time for embedding the needle is no more than two days.

Ⅳ. **Acupuncture with the Electric Needle Apparatuses**

This is a therapeutic technique in which an electric current is applied to the needle which is inserted into the acupoint to strengthen the stimulation on the acupoint. When a needling sensation is induced on the needled part, the needle is charged with a small amount of electrical current. This method combines the needling of the filiform needle with electrical stimulation to achieve curative effects. This electric therapy is not only used in treatment, but also in acupuncture anesthesia for surgical procedures. Its advantages are that it can replace long time sustained manual manipulation of the needle, save manpower and appropriately control the amount of stimu-lation. When the electrical current acts on the human body, the electro-physiological effect can equally produce a therapeutic benefit. This method has a good curative effect on chronic diseases which are difficult to cure because it can bring about a comparatively strong stimulation.

1. **The Selection of the Needle Instruments, Electric Current and Wave Forms**

1) **The Types of Electric Stimulators**

There are different kinds of electric stimulators which can be divided into direct current and alternating current. They can also be classified, on their different structure and functions, as electric stimulators of low-frequency, and high-frequency, of induced and interrupted impulse, of electronic tube, semi-conductor and microwave. All these stimulators have their own advantages and disadvantages.

2) **The Property and Selection of Electric Current**

(1) Smooth Direct Current

When feeding a direct electrical current into the human body, there will be an evident sensation of electrical stimulation. But if continuously used, the stimulated sensation is reduced. The reason for this phenomenon is that part of the current is changed into heat energy and causes electrolysis, electric osmosis and electrophoresis, and the phenomenon of polarization occurs (at the beginning, the current passing through the body tissues is very strong, but if continued, it is reduced). So the disadvantages of using the smooth direct current are that it can bring about burns, or damage the needle due to electrolysis, or cause polarization.

(2) Pulsed Direct Current

The rising and falling edges of this undulating form of pulse current can give the body an obvious stimulation. The function of the middle part of the undulate form is similar to that of the smooth direct current. The electrolysis of the pulsed direct current is more powerful than that of the smooth direct current, so it is usually used as ion implantation.

(3) Alternating Current

The undulate form of this current is composed of normal positive halfwave and negative halfwave. Its stimulation to the human body occurs at the front and back edges of the undulate wave current. The central part of the undulate current produces heat and does not produce electrolysis and polarization, so it is appropriate to be used as the electric needle. But the 50-cycle sine wave of the alternating current is seldom used because of its strong physiological interference to the human body.

(4) Modulated Impulse Current

One kind of impulse wave modulated by another impulse wave with different frequency changes it into a modulated wave. The frequency and the width of the modulated wave varies with the impulse. When the modulated wave stimulates the human body, it can prolong the time it takes for the human body to adapt itself to the electric stimulation.

(5) Mixed Sound and High Frequency Current

When a stimulator with the source from a radio terminal which produces languages, music and noises is used to stimulate the human body, the body cannot adapt itself to it as the amplitude of the wave and the frequency of the current is irregular and varies from time to time. This is its advantage.

In selecting the frequency of electrical stimulation, how the nerves of the human body conduct electrical stimulation should be taken into consideration. The conduction frequency of electrical stimulation through the nerves is usually not more than 2500 times/second. If an electrical impulse with high frequency is used to stimulate the body, part of the electrical energy is wasted as ineffective work since the impulse conduction on the nerves is not more than 2500 times/second, so it is better to design and make an electric stimulator with a circuit producing narrow undulate waves form of oscilation and lower-frequency in order to meet the demands of small size, low power consumption, strong stimulation, safety and low cost.

3) **The Selection of the Undulate Wave Forms of the Pulse Electro-Stimulator and Their Functions**

A brief introduction to the undulate wave forms of the clinically-used electric stimulator and its functions is related as follows:

(1) Dense Wave

Also termed high frequency. Its frequency is high, usually at 50—100 pulses/second. It can reduce nerve irritability. It first produces inhibition on the sensory nerve and then on the motor nerve. This wave(frequency)is usually used to induce analgesic and sedative effects and to relax spasm of both muscles and blood vessels. In addition, it can be applied to anesthesia.

(2) Sparse Wave

Also termed low frequency. Its frequency is low, usually at 2—5 pulses/second. Its stimulation is comparatively strong and can cause contracture of muscles and enhance the tension of muscle and ligaments. Its inhibition on the sensory and motor nerves occurs comparatively late. It is usually used to treat flaccidity, atrophy and the impairment of muscle, joint ligaments and muscle tendons.

(3) Irregular Wave

Also termed alternately dense and sparse wave. This is a kind of undulate wave which results from the spontaneously alternate appearance of low and high waves with a interval time of 1.5 seconds. This kind of wave has an advantage over a single undulate wave which can easily produce adaptability. As applied force is stronger,it has a better excitation effect during treatment and can promote metabolism and blood circulation, improve tissue nutrition and eliminate inflammatory edema. It is usually used to treat sprain and contusion, periarthritis,disturbance of circulation of qi and blood, facial paralysis, myasthenia and local sprain.

(4) Intermittent Wave

This is a rhythmically-interrupted electric wave which occurs automatically. When it stops, there is no impulse output for 1.5 seconds. When it continues, it is a dense wave which works continueously for 1.5 seconds. As its applied force is rather strong, it is not easy for the interrupted undulate wave to cause adaptation in the body, so it can enhance the excitation of muscular tissue and produce good stimulation to the striped muscle and make it contract perfectly. It is usually selected for the treatment of arthralgia syndrome,paralysis, and is also used for electrical muscular stimulation gymnastic training.

(5) Serrated Wave

Also termed sawtooth ware. This is an undulated wave in which impulse wave amplitude undulates automatically in a serrated form 16—20 times or 20—25 times a minute. Its frequency is almost equal to the human respiratory rate,so it is also called respiratory wave and can be used to rescue a person with respiratory failure(whose heart still beats faintly) by making artificial electro-respiration through stimulation of the phrenic nerve(equivalent to Tianding(LI 17)). In addition,it can strengthen the irritability of the nerve and muscle, regulate the functions of meridians and collaterals and improve the circulation of qi and blood.

2. Manipulation and Procedure

1) Selection and Prescription of the Acupoints

Selection of the main and auxilliary acupoints of electric therapy is almost identical to the selection of acupoints of the filiform needle therepy. But the electric therapy must require more than two points each time. Usually it is appropriate to choose 1 to 3 pairs of acupoints on non-homo-lateral sides of the body(i. e. connection of the pairs of points with 1—3 pairs of wires)

Acupuncture selection for electric needling consists of selecting both the acupoints from the area through which the nerve trunk goes and the adjunct acupoints from the local muscular region through which branch nerves run. For example,in the treatment of upper limb paralysis,select Tianding(LI 17) or Quepen(ST 12)(i. e. nerve trunk) as a major point,with Jianliao(SI 14)(i. e. nerve branch) as an adjunct point; or select Quchi(LR 11)(i. e. nerve trunk) as a major point, with Sidu(SJ 9)(i. e. nerve branch)as an adjunct point. In the treatment of lower limb paralysis,take Chongmen(SP 12) or Yinlian(LR 11) (i. e. nerve trunks)as a major point with Jimen(SP 11)(i. e. nerve branch)) as an adjunct points, or select Huantiao(GB 30)(i. e. nerve trunk) as a major point with Weizhong(UB 40)(i. e. nerve branch)as adjunct point. When puncturing major and adjunct acupoints, it is better not to switch on the electric stimulator until the needle response occurs in the affected area. Do not connect too many acupoints each time, otherwise the patient will not be able to stand the strong stimulation or will feel uncomfortable after being needled.

2) Operation of the Electric Stimulation

After obtaining the needling response, do not switch on the electrical power until you have adjusted the output potentiometer of the electric stimulator to "0" and have separately joined the two output wires to the handles or bodies of the two needles. Choose the undulate wave form and frequency and adjust the output current from small to such an extent that the patient can endure it and feel comfortable. It is best to keep the supply on for 10 — 20 minutes. According to the patient's condition, if necessary, the duration of stimulation can be appropriately prolonged. When the treatment is over, turn the output potentiometer back to "0" first, and then switch off the power supply. Remove the wires and finally withdraw the needle as usual. If only one acupoint is needed for the patient's condition, connect one of a pair of leads to the handle of the needle and the other to a thin aluminium plate which is 25cm in size and wrapped by several layers of wet gauze and place it on the skin a little distance from the needle and fasten it with thread. As a result, so obvious is the electric needle response in the needled area, and so concentrated is its stimulation, that any illness may be treated in the needled area. The region of the skin where the aluminium plate is located will not be affected as the induction is very weak and its effect is minor due to the diffusion of the electric current.

3. Indications

Electric needling therapy is almost the same as the filiform needle therapy in its scope of indications. Clinically it is usually used to treat arthralgia-syndrome, flaccidity-syndrome, pain diseases, and induce anesthesia.

4. Precautions

(1) Check the electric stimulator to make sure that its output is normal before each treatment. Turn the output potentiometer back to "0", switch off the power supply and remove the wires after each treatment.

(2) Adjust the flow of the electric current gradually from small to large and take care not to amplify it suddenly in order to prevent strong muscular contracture which would cause unbearable pain to the patient or cause the needle to bend, or break, or the patient to faint.

(3) In treating patients with serious heart disease, take care to prevent the current from going through the heart. When the electric needle is to be applied on the acupoints adjacent to the medullary bulb or the spinal cord, do not use strong electric current stimulation to avoid accidents. Be cautious when applying the electric needle in pregnant women.

(4) If the sensation on one side becomes stronger when the electric needle is applied on symmetrical acupoints on both sides, exchange the two output electrodes with one other. After the exchange has been done, if the stronger sensation becomes weaker, and the weaker sensation becomes stronger, it is the result of the change in the function of the output current of the electric stimulator. If there is no change in sensation, it means that the insertion of the needle is not in the correct anatomical position and should be changed.

(5) The filiform needle which has been burned during the process of moxibustion has lost the capability of conduction due to the oxidation of its handle. Besides, there are other needles which are equally not conductive because of the winding of the needle handle with oxidized golden aluminium wires. When these two kinds of needles are used, connect the electrodes to the shaft of

the needle instead of the handle.

(6) When the electric stimulator is being used, and the output current goes on and off intermittently, it shows that there is something wrong with its output, or the wire is broken or damaged. Do not use it any longer until it is checked and repaired.

(7) When the filiform needle has been used several times, the shaft can easily become defective or damaged. Check the needle carefully before using it to prevent the occurrence of needle breaking.

V. Acupuncture with the Cauterized Needle

This kind of acupuncture is an ancient needling technique in which the acupoints are quickly punctured with a special, non-toxic, stainless needle whose tip is heated red-hot. This gives the patient a stimulation which can warm the meridians to expel the cold, activate blood circulation, remove blood stasis, soften and resolve the hard masses, clear away heat and toxic materials, and elevate the spleen Yang. It can also strengthen the body's resistance to eliminate pathogenic factors, and prevent and cure diseases.

1. The Needle Apparatuses

(1) A thicker stainless needle, such as a sharp ovoid-tip needle or a stainless needle which is 24$^\#$ and 2 cun in length, or sometimes a special-made needle such as a springy cauterized needle which is usually used for superficial treatment, or a rhombold-shaped needle with 18cm in length and a very sharp tip which is used to evacuate the pus from big abscesses.

(2) Burning oil(Chinese bean oil, sesame oil, or castor oil).

(3) A spirit lamp

(4) Sterilized cotton balls and a piece of aseptic gauze.

(5) Adhesive plaster.

2. Manipulation and Procedure

1) Selection and Sterilization of Needling Area

Puncture with a cauterized needle is almost identical to the filiform needle in the selection of acupoints, i. e. selecting acupoints on the basis of an over-all analysis of the illness and the patient's condition. In addition to puncturing the acupoints, needling can also be carried out directly on the affected parts in accordance with various kinds of diseases such as furuncle, flat wart and mole. Generally the points to be punctured should be few, but in case of asthenia symdrome, or in young and middle-aged patients, the number of points can be increased. After the acupoints and locations have been decided upon, sterilization must be carried out. In order to prevent infection, sterilization with 2% iodine tincture and then with 75% alcohol is necessary.

2) Burning of the Needle

Burning the needle is the key step in the application of this kind of needling. The book *Great Compendium on Acupuncture and Moxibustion*(针灸大成, Zhen Jiu Da Cheng) says, "When burning the needle, we must make it red-hot. In this way, the curative effect can be obtained. If the needle is not red hot after heating, it does not produce any beneficial effect on diseases but harms the patients." Therefore, the needle can not be used until it is red-hot when this therapy is administered. A convenient way to make it red-hot is to burn it over a spirit lamp.

3) Puncture and Puncturing Depth

When needling, the clinician must concentrate the mind. Just as the book *Internal Classic*(内经,Nei Jing) says, "Hold the needle as if grasping a tiger and fix your attention upon it in disregard of anything else around. " When puncturing with a cauterized needle, insert the red-hot needle into the selected acupoints quickly and withdraw it immediately. Pay attention to the depth the needle should go. The *Great Compendium on Acupuncture and Moxibustion*(针灸大成,Zhen Jiu Da Cheng) says, "Never puncture too deep for fear that the meridian and vessels should be injured, or too shallow for fear that it should be impossible to cure diseases, so try to puncture not too deep nor too shallow. " The depth of puncture of the cauterized needle is decided according to the cause of illness, the patient's condition and age as well as the thickness of the muscle and the depth of the vessels. Generally speaking, puncture the acupoints on the limbs, waist and abdomen, are deeper, i. e. 0. 2—0. 5 cun; and puncture the acupoints on the chest or back, more shallow, i. e. 0. 1—0. 2 cun.

3. Indications

As pointed out in the *Miraculous Pivot*(灵枢, Ling Shu) "When cauterized needling is used, arthralgia-syndrome can be treated. " The *Great Compendium on Acupuncture and Moxibustion*(针灸大成,Zhen Jiu Da Cheng) says, "It is desirable to evacuate pus from carbuncle or abscess using a cauterized needle. " From these we know that cauterized needle therapy can be used to treat arthralgia-syndrome and evacuate pus from a carbuncle or an abscess. Clinically, the long needle, when inserted deep, is chiefly used to treat scrofulas, furuncles, sores, carbuncles and abscess; while the short needle, when inserted shallow, is used to treat numbness due to pathogenic wind, cold and wetness cold, arthralgia, as well as neurodermatitis and other chronic skin diseases.

4. Precautions

(1) Before application, the practitioner must carefully explain to the patient that cauterized needling does not cause much pain and its therapeutic efficacy is very high to reduce his apprehensions, get rid of the fear of pain and boost the confidence in receiving such treatment.

(2) During the course of puncturing, watch the patient's expression from time to time. If the signs of fainting such as profuse sweating, pale complexion, vomiting and dizziness appear, stop puncturing and withdraw the needle immediately. Let the patient rest in bed and drink some boiled water. If serious, give the patient emergency treatment by puncturing Renzhong(DU 26), Zhongchong(PC 9)and Shixuan(EX —UE 11).

(3) When puncturing, keep the needle away from the vessels and take care not to puncture them, otherwise, an accident may happen.

(4) Be careful when puncturing the points on the face since it is quite possible to leave big scars on the face after cauterized needling. Try not to puncture the points on the face with the exception of treating facial nevi and flat wart.

(5) After needling, in order to prevent local infection, do not wash or bathe till the redness or the swelling, which appears in some locations after puncturing, has subsided.

(6) For the management of the punctured hole. Special treatment is not needed for puncture 0. 1—0. 3 cun deep. If the punctured hole is 0. 4—0. 6 cun deep, dress the hole with a sterilized gauze and fix it with a plaster for 1—2 days to prevent infection.

VI. Pricking, Cutting, Point-Threading, Point-Catgut-Embedding and Point-Ligation Therapies.

The therapies of pricking, cutting and point-threading, point-catgut-embedding and point-ligation are actually the surgical treatment which developed from the theories of meridian and acupoints and has been combined with western medicine.

1. The Pricking Therapy

This method, also called the "root-cutting therapy", is performed by severing the subcutaneous fibre tissue on certain points or area by pricking with a needle or by cutting with a knife. It belonged to the category of blood-letting puncture of ancient times. The *Miraculous Pivot*(灵枢, Ling Shu) says, "The blood vessels…, some of which are as thin as a needle and some of which are larger, if they become very hard and red in color due to swelling, it is necessary to prick them and draw a little blood. "

The area to be pricked can be classified as spot-pricking, acupoint-pricking and division-pricking. The spot-pricking is to prick the red spot or local lesion like node or skin discoloration on certain parts of the skin caused by certain diseases. If there is not a red spot appearing on the skin, the acupoints related to the disease can be pricked, which is called acupoint-pricking. The division-pricking means taking the site related to the disease as the parts to be pricked according to traditional folk experience.

This therapy is applicable for various kinds of diseases, including commonly-encountered and frequently-occurring illnesses. It shows a better therapeutic effect on different sorts of pains, numbness and arthralgia-syndromes. It also has a much better therapeutic effect on certain diseases of the eyes than the other ordinary therapies.

The procedure begins with the preparation of a suture needle, tweezers, sterilized thick silk thread or catgut and an operating knife. Before the operation, get the particular part of the skin to be operated upon sterilized as usual. Insert the needle(if it needs to be threaded, pass a thread through the eye of the needle, approximately 0. 5 cun in length.) horizontally into the skin on the acupoint. After insertion, push and press the skin toward the tip of the needle with the index finger of the left hand and at the same time push in the needle hard with the right hand to make the needle go through the skin. Then, raise the tip a bit and swing the needle side to side slowly several times or whirl the needle slightly a few times to wind the subcutaneous fibre tissue on the end of the needle. Finally, draw the needle out as if sewing with a thread. If the needle carries a thread, pass the thread horizontally through the skin to make the subcutaneous fibre tissue come out with the thread. Break the tissue by cutting it, and keep doing the operation several times until some pieces or all of the white fibre substance has been severed or picked out completely. In addition, 1—2ml of 0. 5% procaine can be administered as local anesthesia. Cutting can also be used instead of pricking. Make an incision 0. 05 cun in length with an operating knife, then pick out the subcutaneous fibre tissues with the tip of the needle. Incise them until all the tissues have been picked out and severed. After the operation, apply a piece of sterilized gauze to the incision and fix it with an adhesive plaster. The operated part can be sterilized with gentian violet and bandaged properly. The needle pricking therapy generally produces a therapeutic effect in a few days (but it will take 30—40 days to produce an effect in the treatment of lymphoid tuberculosis.) If there is no therapeutic effect, prick another point 7—10 days after the first pricking. If the pricking must be done at the same area that has been needled previously, it is necessary to have an interval of 2—3 weeks. The patient should take a lying position while the pricking is being carried out in order to prevent fainting. Local sterilization must be made to prevent infection. It is advisable that the patient not do any heavy physical work or eat a stimulant on the day of the operation. The needle-pricking therapy is contraindicated for pregnant women. It should be used with caution in patients with a tendency to bleed or with hypertension.

2. The Cutting Therapy

This therapeutic technique, also called fat-cutting therapy, is performed by cutting the skin on a particular part of the patient's body with a scalpel to remove a little fatty tissue and give a proper local stimulation. It is particularly used to treat bronchial asthma, chronic bronchitis and other diseases which can be treated with the filiform needle.

The procedure begins with the preparation of a surgical operating knife, a vascular clamp, sterilized gauze, bandage or adhesive plaster,

The parts to be cut are the palm or the acupoints. After the portion is sterilized, give local anaesthesia. Press the lower part of the portion to be cut with the thumb of the left hand and cut through the skin horizontally with an operating knife (not too deep, cutting through the epidermis of the skin will do), the incision being 0.5—1 cun or so in length (shorter for children). After that, separate the incision with straight blood vessel forceps to expose the subcutaneous adipose tissue and take out a piece of adipose tissue as big as a grain of a soybean. Then insert the blood vessel forceps under the skin through the incision and massage by moving the forceps to and fro, up and down to give a strong stimulation until the patient has sensations of aching, swelling and numbness which spreads in all directions. The operator can also grip the subcutaneous or adjacent tissue with the forceps for a few times or slide the blade of the knife on the periosteum (similar to the way of cutting Shanzhong (RN 17)) to make the patient have a strong sensation of pain, fullness and numbness which transmits in a certain direction. It is not necessary to suture the incision after cutting has been done, but it should be bandaged with a sterilized gauze. There is an interval of 7—10 days between two cuttings. Another cutting can be done on either the original acupoint (area) or the new acupoints.

It is important to know whether the patient has a tendency to bleed before cutting. The stimulation should be soft and slight for women, children, the old and the weak. Too much anaesthetic should not be administered. In order not to damage the vessels, nerves and ligaments, the cutting should not go too deep. Sometimes, patients may show various degrees of reaction to the cutting after the operation. Manage or handle the different reactions appropriately. Sterilization must be done to prevent the incision from being infected. The patient should take a good rest, pay particular attention to diet and take good care of oneself.

Besides the pricking and the cutting, there is another therapy called the "scratching therapy", which is to scratch or cut the skin surface or mucosa only.

3. The Point-Threading, Point-Catgut-Embedding and Point-Ligation Therapies

The point-threading, point-catgut-embedding and point-ligation therapies are therapeutic techniques performed by implanting catgut in the meridians and acupoints to serve as a permanent stimulation. They are usually appliable for the treatment of gastric ulcer, duodenal ulcer, sequela of infantile paralysis and asthmatic bronchitis.

The operation begins with commonly-used surgical aseptic procedures: washing the hands, wearing sterile gloves, sterilizing the skin with thiomersalate and spreading an aseptic hole-towel.

1) The Point-Threading Therapy

Perform intracutaneous infiltration anaesthesia with procaine on a spot which is 1. 5—2. 5cm away from the right(or upper) side of the selected acupoint to make a skin cumulus 0. 3—0. 5cm in diameter and on another spot which is 1. 5—2. 5cm away from the left(or lower) side of the acupoint to make another similar skin cumulus. Insert the surgical threaded needle from the skin cumulus on the right(or upper) side, through the deep muscular tissue of the acupoint and draw out the needle from the other skin cumulus on the opposite side(the left or lower). Cut off the catgut on both sides with scissors to prevent infection and make sure the catgut is fully embedded in the skin. Bandage the incision with gauze for 7—9 days.

2) The Point-Catgut-Embedding Therapy

After infiltrating anaesthesia on the selected acupoint with procaine, make an incision on the skin 0. 5—1cm in length with a scalpel. Insert a blood vessel forceps through the fascia, deep into the sensitive spot in the muscular layer beneath the acupoint and massage for a few seconds. After a few minutes, massage around the acupoint once more. The amount of massage is determined in accordance with the state of illness, usually three times or so. Then implant 4—5 pieces of catgut 0. 5—1cm in length in the muscle. The catgut should not be buried superfically in the adipose layer or too deep, this will prevent the catgut from being absorbed or the incision getting infected. Suture the incision with silk thread and bandage it properly with sterilized gauze properly. Remove the silk thread in 5—7 days.

3) The Point-Ligation Therapy

This procedure is similar to that of acupoint threading therapy. It is characterized by the fact that only a small incision is required on the skin cumulus adjacent to the selected acupoint so the anaesthesized skin cumulus is a bit large. First make an incision 0. 3—0. 5cm in length on the surface of the skin cumulus with a sharp and pointed scalpel. Then place a curved hemostat into the deep part of the acupoint and administer a pressure massage. After approximate 40—50 times of flicking stimulation, insert the needle threaded with catgut from the incision to the muscular layer through the deep tissue of the acupoint, then pass the needle through the acupoint and draw the needle out of the incision made on the other skin cumulus on the opposite side of the selected acupoint. After that, immediately insert the same needle to the shallow tissue of the acupoint(the connecting tissue between the muscular layer and the adipose layer) and then draw the needle out from the area where the needle was first inserted. Tighten the two ends of the catgut properly by tying them in a surgical knot and then bury the remaining ends under the skin. Different types of ligation are done according to different conditions . There are various types of ligations such as semicircular ligation, transverse "8" shape ligation, "K" shape ligation and circular ligation . Usually the ligation is made at intervals of 3—4 weeks. If the incision is large, suture the incision with silk thread and bandage it with sterile gauze. Remove the thread in 5—7 days.

Some therapeutic reactions may occur after the therapies of acupoint threading, catgut implantation and ligation. It is normal that the appearance of redness, swelling, heat pain, or even exudation of some fluid on some of the locations is normal and need not be treated. If too much fluid exudes, wipe it away with a sterile cotton ball and bandage it with sterile gauze. Sometimes, general reactions may occur in a few patients, in whom the body temperature increases 4—24 hours after the operation. It will become normal by itself within 2 —4 days.

In addition to that, certain abnormal reactions may occur such as pain, infection of the incisional wound, hemorrhage, or anaphylaxis and nerve injury, so the practitioner must pay close attention to aseptic manipulation when performing such therapies. This therapy is not appliable for patients with serious heart disorders, diabetes or pregnant women. During ligation, attention should be paid to keep clear of vessels and nerves. In the case of paralysis, dirigation (functional training) should be given apart from this treatment.

4. The Acupoint Strong Stimulation Therapy

This is also called "flicking therapy" and is chiefly used to treat muscular paralysis caused by sequela of infantile paralysis and post encephalitis.

Manipulation and Procedure: Select acupoints according to the condition of the patient. The location for the operation is decided according to the different acupoints. After routine sterilization and superficial anaesthesia on the point to be operated with 0.5%—1% procine, cut the skin and subcutaneous tissue open to expose the nerve trunk. Massage the incision with a blood vessel forceps until the patient has a sensation of aching and distending. At this moment, flick the nerve trunk gently with the pointed-tip of the blood vessel forceps for a minute or so. After a little while, resume the flicking for 3—5 times. Suture the incision after the operation and remove the thread after 6—7 days. Advice is to be given to the patient that functional training should start as soon as possible. Give the patient massage and treatment if necessary.

The major acupoints for this therapy: Jianzhen (SI 9), Hegu (LI 4), Huantiao (GB 30), Yanglingquan (GB 34) and Zusanli (ST 36).

Precautions: Since this therapy will produce strong stimulation, it is important for the clinician to explain this to the patient before the operation. The procedure for selecting acupoints is to first choose the acupoints close to the heart, and then those away from the heart. The local anaesthesia should not be too deep and the manipulation should be gentle and dexterous. Watch closely the response of the patient during the operation.

VII. Hydro-Acupuncture(Point-Injection) Therapy

Hydro-acupuncture therapy is a treatment which combines acupuncture with medicine. Based on the meridian theories, Chinese or Western medicines are selected and injected into a relevant acupoint, pressure-pain point or positive reaction point. These are found by palpation on the body surface so as to modulate the function of the body and treat diseases through the combined action of acupuncture and medicine.

1. Manipulation and Procedure

Find the clearly positive reactive Back-shu points and Front-Mu points along the lines of their distribution. Or based on the principle of common prescriptions in acupuncture therapy, select the main acupoints corresponding with the diseases. After routine sterilization, puncture the skin quickly with a syringe needle. Then, manipulate it slowly and insert the needle accurately into the acupoint or the positive reaction point. After the patient has a sensation of aching and distending, pull the stylet up a little bit. If no blood comes out, inject the liquid medicine. To treat common diseases, the speed of injection should be medium. Since patients with chronic diseases or in poor health usually require a slight stimulation, the medicine should be injected slowly. On the contrary, the patients with acute diseases or with a strong body usually require a strong stimulation. The medicine should be injected quickly. If more liquid medicine needs to be injected, the injection can be given with the gradual withdrawing of the syringe from the deep to the superficial muscular layer, or inject the medicine in different directions. The amount of liquid medicine injected each time in each acupoint varies from 0.3—0.5ml for the acupoints on the head, face and ears to 2—15ml for the acupoints on the four limbs and the back where the muscles are thick. The amount can be increased or reduced according to the state of illness or the different concentration of the liquid medicine. The choice of the solution should be made according to the condition of the patient. Generally the traditional Chinese and western medicines which are suitable for intramuscular injection are 5%— 10% glucose, normal saline, water, vitamin B1 B12, all kinds of tissue fluid, procaine as well as the water extract of Danggui(Radix Angelicae Sinensis), Chuanxiong(Rhizoma Ligustici Chuanxiong), and Honghua(Flos Carthami). The puncture can be carried out once a day or every other day, 7—12 times constituting a course. An interval of 3— 5 days is allowed between two courses.

2. Indications

It is appliable for various kinds of painful diseases and soft tissue injury and contusion which include pain in the loin and legs, aching of shoulder and back, arthralgia, sciatica, scapulohumeral periarthritis, lumbar muscle sprain, fibrositis, benign arthritis as well as bronchitis, hypertension, gastric ulcer, duodenal ulcer, hepatitis, biliary colic, neurosism and sequela of concussion of the brain.

3. Precautions

It is necessary to explain to the patient the characteristics and post-reactions of this therapy such as sensations of aching, swelling or heat on the injected portion to eliminate the patient's worries. Pay close attention to the asepic precautions to prevent infection. Take notice of the properties of medicine being used. Medicine is capable of producing allergic reaction, therefore a skin test should be made. For those who receive such treatment for the first time, or the aged and the weak patients, use fewer acupoints for injection and reduce the quantity of injection. Do not make an injection in the lumbosacral area for pregnant women. In principle, do not inject liquid medicine into the articular cavity in order to avoid redness, swelling and aching on the joints. Never use hypertonic glucose in the subcutaneous layer, but only in the intramuscular.

Appendix   Air Acupuncture(Point-Injection) Therapy

This is a therapeutic technique characterized by injecting sterilized air into certain acupoints with a syringe. It regulates the function of the meridian by stimulation produced through the injected air which makes a "cavity" for some time before it is completely absorbed.

(1) Manipulations and Procedure

After sterilizing the skin over the acupoint, cover the tip of syringe with a sterile cotton ball and fill the syringe with the filtered air, then, immediately insert the needle into the acupoint to the required depth. When the needling sensation appears, draw the plunger up a bit to see if blood comes out. If no blood appears, inject the air slowly(3—5ml in one acupoint each time). After completing the injection, withdraw the syringe, cover and press the punctured hole with a dry sterile cotton ball and rub it gently for a while. The injection can be done every other day or every two days.

(2) Precautions

Make sure that the needle of the syringe is not in a blood vessel when injecting air so as to prevent the occurrence of air embolic diseases due to the entering of air into the vessels.

Chapter Four

General Introduction to Moxibustion Therapy

Moxibustion was called "Rui(灬)" in ancient times. The Dictionary of *Shuo Wen Jie Zi*(说文解字,Shuo Wen Jie Zi) says, "Moxibustion means burning and is a therapeutic method that an ignited moxa is placed close to the human body to warm the local area." Ancient people applied the ignited moxa to treat diseases by warming certain parts of the body. For thousands of years, other materials such as an oil lamp,sulphur and drugs were also applied. Moxa has long been used as the main material for moxibustion.

I. Moxibustion Classification and Its Commonly Used Materials

1. Moxibustion Classification

Moxibustion has been used to treat diseases for thousands of years. At first there was a simple form of moxa moxibustion, and later, it evolved into various types of moxibustion. Generally, moxibustion can be divided into two types: the moxa moxibustion and non-moxa moxibustion, of which, the moxibustion with moxa cone and moxa stick are the most commonly used. When administering moxibustion, the method of putt ing the ignited moxa cone directly over an acupoint on the skin is termed direct moxibustion,also named apparent moxibustion; the method of placing the moxa cone on a slice of ginger, garlic, or on a small amount of salt, or on a herbal cake before igniting, it is termed indirect moxibustion, also called separation moxibustion.

Classification of moxibustion is as follows: (See Fig. 4—1)

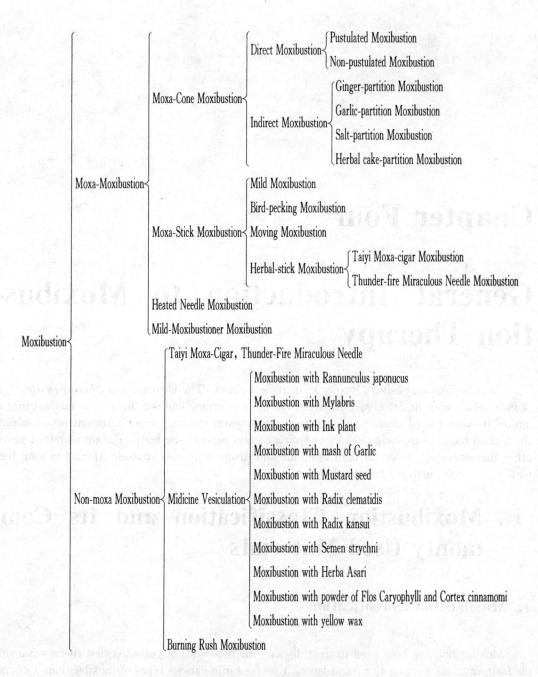

Fig. 4－1 Classification of Moxibustion

2. Commonly Used Materials for Moxibustion

In the beginning, only moxa was used for moxibustion, other materials were incorporated later.

Different materials are chosen for different types of moxibustion. Moxa, made of dry mugwort leaves, is the commonly used raw material today. *Compendium of Materia Medica*（本草纲

目，Ben Cao Gang Mu) says，"Mugwort leaves can be used for many kinds of diseases. " *New Compilation of Materia Medica*(本草从新，Ben Cao Cong Xin) says，"Mugwort leaves are bitter and acrid in flavor，warm and hot in nature after preparation. It has a pure Yang property and can recuperate the depleted Yang and restore consciousness to the patient. It can travel all the twelve meridians，treat all Yin syndromes，regulate Qi and blood，dispel cold and dampness evils，and warm the uterine cavity⋯. Moxibustion can dredge all the meridians and eliminate hundreds of diseases. " The processed soft dry mugwort floss has the following special advantages：

1) It is convenient to make moxa cones in different sizes，and the mugwort flow is inflammable with a fragrant smell.

2) The mild heat it produces can penetrate the skin and warm the deep parts of the body. Since its raw material，Folium Artemislae，is distributed in most parts of China，it is easy to obtain.

The fresh thick leaves are gathered every May. They are dried in sunlight，pounded into pieces after the stalks，mud and sand are removed by sieving. They are dried and pounded again several times，and finally the slightly yellow-coloured soft mugwort floss is made. According to the different processing(pounding) used，the mugwort floss may be divided into several grades. Generally the fine moxa is used for direct moxibustion and the thick，rough one for indirect moxibustion. The longer the floss is preserved，the better effect it has. The mugwort floss should be kept in a dry container to avoid turning moistened and mildewed.

The moxa materials sold in today's market are moxa granules，moxa cones，non-smoking moxa cones and small moxa cones.

II. Functions of Moxibustion

In moxibustion therapy，the most commonly used is the moxibustion with moxa floss. The function of moxibustion，apart from warming and heating stimulation，is concerned with the property of the argyi leaves. *New Compilation of Material Medica*(本草从新，Ben Cao Cong Xin) says，"Argyi leaves are bitter，acrid in flavor，warm and pure Yang in nature and can recuperate the depleted Yang. It can travel the twelve meridians，regulate Qi and blood，despel cold-dampness，warm the uterine cavity，⋯ the heat produced by moxibustion can dredge all the meridians to eliminate diseases. " What the above indicates is that the argyi leaves，as the moxibustion material，have many therapeutic effects descibed below：

1. Warming and Dispersing the Cold Evil

Moxibustion can disperse cold evil by the heat produced by moxa floss and other materials. It is effective for cold syndromes including asthenia due to cold evil and general cold syndrome due to Yang deficiency. Just as *Plain Questions*(素问，Su Wen)says，"Qi and blood are inclined towards warming instead of cooling，Stagnations of the Qi and blood caused by cold evil can be relieved by heat. "

2. Warming and Dredging the Meridians，and Promoting Blood Circulation to Remove Blood Stasis.

Heat stimulation by moxibustion can warm the meridians and collaterals and also promote the flow of Qi and blood. Therefore it can be used for stagnation syndromes of Qi and blood and blockage of the meridians and collaterals due to exogenous evils，such as wind-cold-dampness type of arthralgia.

3. Recuperating the Depleted Yang and Rescuing Collapsed Patients

Moxibustion can warm and reinforce Yang syndrome due to depleted Yang including profuse perspiration, coldness of the extremities and indistinct pulse which can be treated by frequent and heavy moxibustion. Collapsing syndromes such as enuresis, prolapse of rectum, and hysteroptosis due to Yang deficiency can also be treated by moxibustion.

4. Relieving Stagnation and Dispersing Accumulated Evil

Qi is the commander of blood and blood flows following the Qi. So if Qi flows unobstructedly, blood can circulate normally. Qi travels faster when it is heated. Since moxibustion can smooth the circulation of Qi and blood, relieve stagnation and disperse accumulated evils, it is often used for mastitis in early stage. It is also used for scrofula and cold pyogenic infection which has not yet festered.

5. Preventing Diseases and Promoting Health

Moxibustion has long been a method for tonification among the people. *Thousands of Golden's Priscriptions*(千金方, Qian Jin Fang) says "Do moxibustion on the body to avoid malaria." *Experiences of Bianque*(扁鹊 心书, Bian Que Xin Shu) says, "Frequent moxibustion on Guanyuan(RN4), Qihai(RN 6), Mingmen(DU 4) and Zhongwan(RN 12) will prolong a person's life to a hundred years." These two quotations indicate that moxibustion can excite the vital qi, reinforce the capacity of resisting against diseases to attain the purpose of preventing diseases. Just like the saying goes, "To stay healthy, frequently perform moxibustion on Zusanli (ST 36)."

III. Precautions for Moxibustion

1. Body Position for Moxibustion

Just like with acupuncture, a proper position should be chosen in doing moxibution. For example, sit upright when the moxibustion is done at the acupoints below the knees. During moxibustion, the position should be natural with the muscle relaxed. Direct moxibustion must be done many times, so it is important to locate acupoints precisely at the first time. If the point is located incorrectly, correct it as soon as possible.

2. General Procedure of Moxibustion

Moxibustion is usually done on the Yang meridians first, then on the Yin meridians; on the upper parts of the body first, then the lower parts. That is, using the acupoints on the back first, then those on the chest and abdomen; the acupoints on the head and body first, then those on the four extremities. However, in a clinic, the procedure should vary with the different conditions of the patients.

3. Quantity of Moxibustion

Burning one moxa cone is called one "Zhuang(壮)". There are three types of moxa cones in different sizes. Small or moderate cones are usually applied for direct moxibustion, and moderate or large ones for indirect moxibustion. In clinic, the quantity of moxibustion is computed by the size and number of the cones, and its use varies with the need of different constitutions, diseases and sites of the patient. More cones can be used on the lumbar, back and abdomen, less on the chest and four extremities, and even less on the head and neck. More cones are used on adults which requires a long time; less cones on the old and children which rquires a short time. Generally, moxibustion with moxa-stick and warming moxibustion is computed by the burning time, while the Taiyi Moxa-cigar and Thunder-fire Miraculous moxihustions are computed by the number of manipulations.

4. Management of the Moxibustion Scar

Vesiculations, scabs and ulcers sometimes can be caused by direct moxibustion. If these happen, they can be managed by covering them with antiseptics, dressings or adhesive plasters to prevent contamination or infection. For small ulcers, just have it scab on its own and no treatment is needed. Reddish skin and heat sensation may disappear by themselves soon after moxibustion.

5. Contraindication for Moxibustion

A. Moxibustion can reinforce Yang and also reduce Yin, so it is contraindicated for the diseases which manifest as Yin deficiency and Yang hyperactivity and also for the patients with invasion of the interior of the body by pathogenic heat. Care should be taken when treating such diseases as consumptive illness due to Yin deficiency, hemoptysis, headache, excessive noxious heat due to excess of liver Yang and asthenia type coma resulting from apoplexy.

B. Direct moxibustion is prohibited on the face, pudendum and the area where the main blood vessels lie. Moxibustion cannot be used on the abdomen and lumbosacral regions of a pregnant woman.

C. Today, fewer acupoints are contraindicated for moxibustion than those recorded in the ancient texts. The prohibited acupoints are Jingming(BL 1), Sizhukong(SJ 23), Tongziliao(GB 1), Renying(ST 9), Jingqu(LU 8), Quze(PC 3)and Weizhong(BL 40). In addition, attention shold be paid to patients with an insensible feeling, numbness of the extremities or one who may faint so as to avoid scalding them.

Chapter Five

Special Introduction to Moxibustion Therapy

In this chapter, several commonly used manipulations of moxibustion in clinic are introduced. In Chinese medicine, different types of moxibustion and different moxibustion areas should be chosen according to different kinds of diseases and syndromes. When the method changes, the function(reinforcing or reducing)also changes.

I. Moxibustion with Moxa Cone

There are two types of moxa cone moxibustion, the direct moxibustion and indirect moxibustion. Moxa cone is shaped like a circular cone made of dry moxa floss. Generally, for direct moxibustion a small cone is used, and for indirect moxibustion a large one is often used. When one cone is burned out, it means finishing one "Zhuang(壮)". (Fig. 5—1)

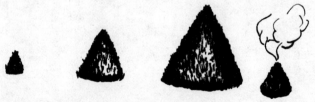

Fig. 5—1 Moxa Cones

Moxa cone is made by kneading the floss with fingers into the shape of a grain or a cone. For direct moxibustion, the circular moxa cones, which are made of extremely fine floss in a grain size, are ignited directly on the acupoints of the skin. Moxa cones made of rough floss, in a broad bean or soybean size, should be burned on a slice of ginger, garlic or on a herbal cake for indirect moxibustion. For heated-needle moxibustion, the floss is round and pressed, shaped and sized like a jujube-pit. It is then encircled around the handle of a filiform needle and is ignited. Today it is more convenient to use the moxa cones which are pressed and processed by special machinery. The size and the number of the moxa cones to be used are influenced by many factors such as body constitution, course or condition of the disease, location of the acupoint, function of reinforcing or reducing, climate, and whether the patient has received this kind of therapy before, or whether the operator wants to make the skin fester or not. *Great Compendiums on Acupuncture and Moxibustion*(针灸大成, Zhen Jiu Da Cheng)says, "To reinforce, avoid blowing the fire, let the cone burn out by itself, and then press the acupoint; To reduce, blow at the ignited cone, to make it burn quickly and do not press the acupoints. " In the clinic, moxibustion can reinforce the deficiency by having the ignited moxa cones burn out slowly by themselves to get a comparatively long-time mild heat, and then pressing the acupoint with fingers to gather the Qi. It can also purge the evils of the excess syndromes by blowing at the ignated cone to quicken its burning out in a short time. After that, don't press the acupoints to disperse evils.

1. Direct Moxibustion

There are two types of direct moxibustion, the pustule-forming moxibustion and non-pustule-forming moxibustion. (Fig. 5－2)

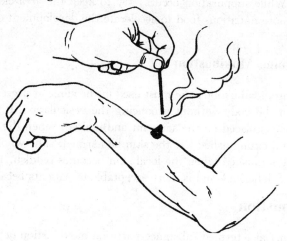

Fig. 5－2 Direct Moxibustion

1) Pustule-Forming Moxibustion

Pustule-forming moxibustion is also called scar moxibustion. It is a direct moxibustion method of burning a moxa cone in the size of a grain on the skin to produce local vesiculation and then aseptic suppuration. Therapeutic effects are gained in this way in improving the body constitution and reinforcing the resistance against diseases. *Experience on Acupuncture and Moxibustion* (针灸资生经, Zhen Jiu Zi Sheng Jing) says, "The diseases will be cured if a scar appears after the moxibustion. " So, in ancient times, the occurrence of the scar indicated a therapeutic effect and was often regarded as the key to the obtaining of curative effect. Today, this method is applicable to asthma, chronic tracheitis, chronic gastrointestinal diseases, poor body constitution and underdevelopement.

Procedures:

(1) Body Position and Location of the Acupoints

Select a proper, comfortable and flat position which can be kept for a long period. Then locate the acupoints and mark them with mercurochrome or gentian violet if necessary. *Thousands of Golden Priscriptions*(千金方, Qian Jin Fang)says, "Keep the extremities flat and straight instead of bending them. Keep a sitting posture if the acupoints have been located in a sitting position and keep a lying posture after locating the acupoints in a lying position." It shows that ancient people paid much attention to the body position and location of acupoints for moxibustion.

(2) Fixing the Moxa Cones and Igniting.

When moxa cones are made from fine mugwort floss, in order to promote the permeability of the heating, some fragrant herbal powders such as Clove(丁香, Ding Xiang), Cortex Cinnamomi(肉桂, Rou Gui) can be added into. Spread garlic fluid or vaseline on the acupoints to increase the stickiness and the stimulation before igniting the cones. When the patient feels burning pain, the operator may pat the skin around the acupoint to reduce the pain. Clean the acupoint with a gauze soaked in sterile water after one cone is finished. Change a new cone to continue the course. Generally, 5—9 cones are used on each acupoint.

(3) Applying the Herbal Plaster

Apply the herbal plaster on the acupoints after the moxibustion is over and change a new one daily. Aseptic suppuration will happen on the acupoints several days later. Change the plaster frequently if there is much pus. The moxibustion sore will scab and crust after 30—40 days, and then a scar may form. While suppuration occurs, try to keep the area clean to avoid infection. The patient should eat more nutritious food to accelerate the development of the sore so as to enhance the curative effect.

2) Non-Pustule-Forming Moxibustion

Non-pustule-forming moxibustion, the most used in the clinic at present, is a method by using moxa cones to warm the body without producing the vesiculation. It is also called non-scar moxibustion. A small cone is placed on the acupoint and ignited. When the patient feels pain, the moxa cone is removed and extinguished lest the skin be harmed. The whole procedure uses 3—7 cones for each point and is finished when the local skin becomes reddish. This method is applicable for cold syndromes of deficiency and is more acceptable to patients because of its non-scaring.

2. Indirect Moxibustion

Indirect moxibustion, also termed substance-partition moxibustion or partition moxibustion, is performed by placing some materials, usually drugs, between the smoldering moxa cone and the skin. This method serves as the treatment of both moxibustion and drugs at the same time. Since this kind of moxibustion does not require plister and purulence, patients are usually willing to accept it. Commonly used indirect moxibustion in clinic includes the following:

1) Ginger-Partition Moxibustion

In this method, a slice of ginger is used to seperate the ignited moxa cone and the skin. Ginger(生姜, Sheng Jiang), which has an acrid taste and a warm nature, can lift Yang and disperse stagnated energy, regulate the Qi of Ying and Wei, expel cold evil and dredge the meridians and collaterals. It is effective for diseases due to wind evil and cold-dampness evil. Applying both fresh ginger and moxa can avoid scarring and has a dual therapeutic effect. Cut a slice of ginger about 0.2 cun thick, punch several small holes at its center, place it on the acupoint selected. Then, place a large moxa cone on the ginger and ignite it for moxibustion. When the patient complains of burning pain, some dry cotton or thick paper can be placed below the ginger slice.

Stop the moxibustion until there is a local erythema of the skin. This type of moxibustion is easy to use and usually does not scald the patient. (See Fig. 5—3)

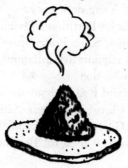

Fig. 5—3   Ginger-Partition Moxibustion

Ginger-partition moxibustion is mainly applicable for syndrome of deficiency such as abdominal pain, diarrhea, vomiting, nocturnal emission due to deficiency of kidney, Bi-syndrome due to wind-cold-dampness evil and flaccidity of extremities.

2) Garlic-Partition Moxibustion

Garlic, with an acrid taste and warm nature, can eliminate swellings, disperse accumulated evils, draw out pus and relieve pains. Cut a slice of raw one-head garlic about 0. 1 cun thick, punch several small holes in the center and place it on the acupoint or on the swelling area. Then, place the moxa cone on the garlic and ignite it for moxibustion. After 4—5 cones are burned, replace the garlic with another one and continue. At each acupoint, burn 5—7 cones totally. Since the juice of garlic is a stimulate to the skin, there may appear vesiculation after moxibustion. *Thousands Golden Prescriptions*(千金方, Qian Jin Fang) indicates that garlic-partition moxibustion is effective for scrofula and suppurative inflammation of the skin. *The Golden Mirror of Medicine*(医宗金鉴, Yi Zong Jin Jian) and *Elementary of Medicine*(医学入门, Yi Xue Ru Men) say that it can treat carbuncle and pyogenic infection of the skin. Today, in the clinic, it is mainly used for lung-deficiency tuberculosis, mass in the abdomen, pyogenic infections and an abscess which has not festered.

3) Salt-Partition Moxibustion

Salt-partition moxibustion is also termed Moxibustion at Shenque (RN 8) because it is applied only at the point of Shenque(RN 8). To apply, fill the umbilicus with salt to the level of the skin, place the moxa cone on a slice of ginger or directly on the salt and ignite it for moxibustion. The use of ginger prevents the patient from being scalded, which may be caused by the explosion of the heated salt. This method is very effective for acute abdominal pain, vomiting, diarrhea, dysentery, cold extremities and collapse syndromes. In addition, it has the function of recuperating the depleted Yang and rescuing unconscious patients.

4) Herbal Cake-Partition Moxibustion

(1) Monkshood(附子, Fu Zi)-Partition Moxibustion

Use a piece of Monkshood or a monkshood cake as the partition. Then, punch numerous holes in its centre and place it on the acupoint selected. Then place a moxa cone on it and ignite the cone for moxibustion. The monkshook cake is made by grinding the mondshood into a paste, mix it with yellow rice wine and make into a cake 2—3 cun thick. Since this herb has an acrid taste and is extremely hot in nature, it has the function of warming the kidney and activating Yang. So it is often used for all kinds of diseases of Yang deficiency.

（2）Semen Sojao Preparatum（豆豉，Dou Chi）Cake-Partition Moxibustion

The cake is made by mixing the powder of Semen Sojao Preparatum with yellow rice wine. It is used for carbuncle and various chronic stubbon suppurative inflammations.

（3）Pepper（胡椒，Hu Jiao）Cake-Partition Moxibustion

The cake is made of a mixture of white pepper and flour, about the thickness of a coin. The center of the cake is depressed to fill the powders of Clove（丁香，Ding Xiang），Musk Moschus（麝香，She Xiang）and Cortex Cinnamomi（肉桂，Rou Gui）. The moxa cone is fixed on the cake and then ignited for moxibustion. This type of moxibustion is used for Bi-syndromes（arthralgia）due to wind-cold-dampness and local numbness.

II. Moxibustion with Moxa Stick

The moxa stick is made in the following way:

Spread 24g of pure and soft floss on a piece of soft and good quanlity mulberry or cotton paper（26×20cm）, roll the paper into a cylinder as tightly as possible with a diameter of 1.5 cm and seal it with glue. If the moxa stick is made with a mixture of herbal powders and mugwort floss, it is drug-moxa stick. The moxa-stick moxibustion is classified as the mild-warm moxibustion, sparrow-pecking moxibustion and rounding moxibustion.（See Fig. 5—4）

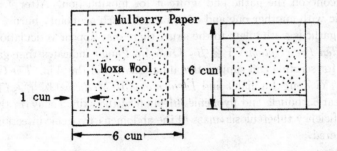

Fig. 5—4   Moxa Sticks

1. Mild-Warming Moxibustion

Ignite one end of the moxa stick, hold the stick and keep the ignited end 0.5—1.0 cun above the selected acupoint without moving, and heat the area for 3—5 minutes each time. The treatment stops when there is a local erythema of the skin. The sensation should be a local warming sensation instead of burning pain. The moxibustion temperature may be checked or controlled by placing the index and middle fingers on the skin when the patient is a child, or he or she is in coma, or the local parts of his or her body is insensitive to heat（See Fig. 5—5）.

2. Sparrow-Pecking and Rounding Moxibustions

By calling it sparrow-pecking, it means holding an ignited moxa stick with its ignited end di-

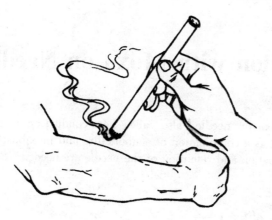

Fig. 5—5   Mild-Warming Moxibustion

rectly at the acupoint and moving it up and down, like a bird pecking food. (See Fig. 5—6)
Rounding moxibustion, also termed circling moxibustion, involves keeping the ignited moxa stick
above the selected acupoint, and moving the stick in a circular fashion horizontally and repeatedly
meanwhile. (See Fig. 5—7)

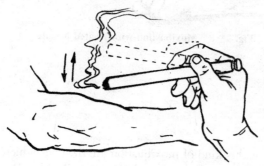

Fig. 5—6   "Sparrow-Pecking" Moxibustion

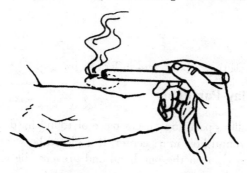

Fig. 5—7   Circling Moxibustion

Different methods and heating time of moxibustion determine whether it is reinforcing or
reducing. Modern acupuncturist Zhulian is of the opinion that mild-warming or rounding moxibustion, if it is used at one point for more than ten minutes, has an inhibitory action and can
calm the mind and relieve pain which is similar to the reducing method in acupuncture therapy.
Sparrow-pecking moxibustion, if it is used at one point for 0.5 to 2 minutes and 30—50 times,
or if the mild-warming moxibustion and rounding moxibustion are conducted at one point for only
3—5 minutes, has an exciting action and can promote physiological function and relieve restraint
which is similar to the reinforcing method in acupuncture therapy.

Ⅲ. Moxibustion with Moxa on Needle

Moxibustion with moxa on needle, also called heat-conducting moxibustion and burned needle-handle moxibustion, is a combination of acupuncture and moxibustion. It is used for diseases in which both moxibustion and retention of the needle are needed. (See Fig. 5—8)

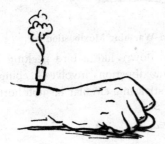

Fig. 5—8　Moxibustion with Heated Needle

1. Apparatuses

1) Filiform Needles

Filiform needles used for this kind of moxibustion are the ones which are applied in acupuncture therapy in the clinic. It is better to remove the needle tail. In order to reduce the resistance of fixing the moxa section to the handle of the needle, it is recommended that the needle whose handle is coiled not be used.

2) Moxa Sections

Moxa sticks are cut into sections about 2cm in length for use.

3) Temperature-Controlling Partition

For a temperature-controlling partition, use a piece of round hard cardboard approximately 5cm in diameter with a small round hole in its center. It is placed between the moxa cone and the acupoint to reduce the burning pain on the one hand and prevent the ignited moxa from falling down to burn the skin on the other.

4) Heated-Needle Fork

The heated-needle fork is made of 6—8 strands of 16# iron wires which are twisted together. Ignite the moxa sections which has been fixed on the fork. Then place the fork together with ignited moxa sections to the handle of the needle which had been inserted into the acupoints. In this way, more heat from the moxa sections is gained and an accident due to fallen moxa is avoided. Generally the therapeutic effect is improved by applying only one time of moxibustion.

2. Manipulation and Procedures

This kind of moxibustion is the combination of acupuncture and moxibustion. After reinforcing or reducing the manipulation of acupuncture, retain the needle at the proper depth. Fix the moxa section around the handle of the needle and ignite the moxa. Indirect heated needle moxibustion requires a partition between the moxa and the skin, while direct heated needle moxibustion does not.

1) Direct Heated Needle Moxibusiton

Ignite the low end of the moxa section which has been fixed on the needle handle; or cover the acupoint with a temperature-controlled partition before the moxa section is fixed on the needle, then ignite the moxa. The number of moxa sections used varies with the condition of the patient.

2) Indirect Heated Needle Moxibustion

(1) Ginger-Partition Heated Needle Moxibustion

Cut a slice of raw ginger about 2—3mm thick, punch several holes at its center, place it on the skin with the needle passing through its center. Then place the moxa section onto the needle handle. The number of moxa section used varies with the condition of the patient.

(2) Garlic-Partition Heated Needle Moxibustion

Cut a slice of raw one-head garlic 2—3mm thick, punch several holes in its center, place it on the skin with the needle passing through its center. Then place the moxa section onto the needle handle. The number of moxa sections used varies with the condition of the patient.

3) Indications

This method is applicable for cold-syndromes such as rheumatism, joint aches, numbness, diarrhea and distention of the abdomen due to deficiency and cold.

Commonly used acupoints for heated needle moxibustion include the acupoints of the 14 meridians and some extra acupoints, of which the most commonly used are the Jiaji points and the back-shu points of the Bladder Meridian.

4) Precautions

(1) The patient should maintain a proper body position and try not to shift the body to prevent the occurrence of a bent or broken needle, or removal of the moxa.

(2) Before heating the needle, the operator should explain to the patient about the superiority and safety of this method and encourage the patient to relax to avoid fainting during moxibustion. The supine or prone position are prefered.

(3) If the patient feels chilly and suffers from convulsions, the operator should check the room temperature. Usually this ease is caused by the low temperature of the room. The operator should withdraw the needle and try to raise the temperature. Have the patient drink hot water and spread hot towels over the limbs to warm and calm the patient.

(4) During the moxibustion, if the patient receives a burn, it can be treated in the same manner as a moxibustion sore.

Ⅳ. Moxibustion with Instruments

1. Apparatus

Moxibustion with instruments, also called mild-container moxibustion, is actually a kind of hot medicated compress. The instruments are metal containers used to hold the moxa and medicine with numerous small openings on the botton. (See Fig. 5－9).

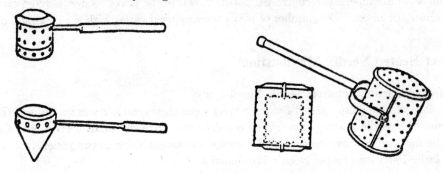

Fig. 5－9 The Articles of Moxibustioners

2. Manipulation and Procedure

When this moxibustion is conducted, put the moxa and drugs in the instrument and ignite them. Then, place and move it about on the desired region. It is suitable for women, children and individuals who are apprehensive about conventional moxibustion therapy.

Ⅴ. Other Types of Moxibustions

1. Taiyi Moxa-Cigar and Thunder-Fire Miraculous Moxibustion

1) Taiyi Moxa-Cigar Moxibustion

(1)Preparation of the Moxa-Cigar
The ingredients are:
Ginseng(人参,Ren Shen)120g
Notoginseng(参三七,Shen San Qi)240g
Blood of goat(山羊血,Shan Yang Xue)60g
Rhizoma Homalomenae(千年健,Qian Nian Jian)480g

Cortex Schizo phragmatis Integrifolii Radicis(钻地风,Zuan Di Feng)480g

Cassia Bark(肉桂,Rou Gui)480g

Pericarpium Zanthoxyli(川椒,Chuan Jiao)480g

Olibanum(乳香,Ru Xiang)480g

Myrrha(没药,Mo Yao)480g

Squama Manitis(穿山甲,Chuan Shan Jia)240g

Fennel Fruit(小茴香,Xiao Hui Xiang)480g

Rhizoma Atractylodis(苍术,Cang Zhu)480g

Moxa(蕲艾,Qi Ai)1920g

Liquorice Root(甘草,Gan Cao)960g

Radix Ledebouriellae(防风,Fang Feng)1920g

Musk(麝香,She Xiang) a bit

Grind the above into powders. Spread appropriate amount of pure and soft moxa on a piece of cotton paper(40×40cm), and mix it with 24g of the herbal powders. Then roll the paper tightly into a stick just like a firecraker. Wrap the stick with mulberry paper again, and dry it in the shade for future use.

(2) Procedures

Ignite one end of the stick, wrap the burning end with seven layers of coarse cloth and press it immediately on the acupoints or the area to be treated. When the stick cools, do the same procedure again. The treatment should be repeated 5—7 times on each acupoint or the area. This Taiyi Moxa-cigar is used to treat wind-cold-dampness arthralgia, various pains and hemiplegia due to flaccidity syndrome.

2) **Thunder-Fire Miraculous Moxibustion**

(1) Preparation of the Moxa Roll

The ingredients are:

Folium Artemisiae Argyi(艾绒,Ai Rong) 90g

Eagle Wood(沉香,Chen Xiang) 9g

Radix Aucklamdiae(木香,Mu Xiang) 9g

Olibanum(乳香,Ru Xiang) 9g

Herba Artemisiae Scopariae(茵陈,Yin Chen) 9g

Rhizoma Seu Radix Notopterygii(羌活,Qiang Huo)

Dried Ginger(干姜,Gan Jiang) 9g

Squama Manitis(穿山甲,Chuan Shan Jia) 9g

Musk(麝香,She Xiang) a bit

(2) Procedures

Grind the above into powders. Spread the moxa on a piece of cotton paper and mix the powders with the moxa. Then roll the paper tightly into a stick like a firecracker. Finally coat the stick with the egg white, wrap and seal it with mulberry for 6—7 times and dry it in the shade. The operation and function of this kind of Thunder-Fire Miraculous Moxibustion is almost the same as the Taiyi Moxa-cigar moxibustion.

2. **Crude Herb Moxibustion**

This method, also called medicinal vesiculation or medical blister moxibustion, is a therapy in which irritative drugs are applied on the acupoints so as to cause blisters. The commonly used materials in this moxibustion are as follows:

Ranunculus japonucus(毛茛,Mao Lang) Moxibustion

Mash the leaves well and plaster the paste on Cunko. The following day, a blister will appear. If it is heated with fire, it can treat malaria.

Mylabris(斑蝥，Ban Mao) Moxibustion

Put the Mylabris in the vinegar and use the soaked Mylabris to rub the affected part. It can treat psoriasis, neurodermatitis and arthralgia.

Ink plant(旱莲草，Han Lian Cao) Moxibustion

Mash the herb well and apply the paste to the acupoint to make the area blister. This method is used in treating malaria.

Garlic (蒜泥，Suan Ni) Moxibustion

Apply the garlic paste to the acupoint of Yuji(LU 10)in Taiyin Meridian of the hand to cause blistering. It is used for inflammation of the throat.

Mustard seed(白芥子，Bai Jie Zi)Moxibustion

Grind the seeds into powder and apply it on the skin to cause local congestion and vesiculation. This method is primarily used for Yin cellulitis, subcutaneous nodule, swelling and pain in the knee.

Radix Clematidis root (威灵仙，Wei Ling Xian) Moxibustion

Mash the fresh leaves into paste and apply it on the skin externally. It is often used to treat hemorrhoids(Zusanli(ST 36)), acute conjunctivitis(Taiyang(EX-HN5)), pertussis(Shenzhu (DU 12)) and tonsillitis (Tianrong(SI 17)).

Kansui root (甘遂，Gan Sui) Moxibustion

Grind the herb into powder and apply it on the skin. It can treat malaria(Dazhui(DU 14)), asthma(Feishu(BL 13)) and uroschesis(Zhongji (RN 3)).

Semen Strychni (马钱子，Ma Qian Zi) Moxibustion

The herb is ground into powder and applied on Jiache(ST 6) and Dicang(ST 4); treating facial paralysis.

Herb Asari(细辛，Xi Xin) Moxibustion

The herb is ground into powder, mixed with vinegar and applied externally. If it is applied on Yongquan(KI 1) or Shenque(RN 8), it treats infantile stomatitis.

Cloves and Cassia bark(丁香，肉桂，Ding Xiang and Rou Gui)Moxibustion

Grind the both into powder and fill the umbilicus with the powder. It can treat diarrhea of children.

Yellow Wax (黄蜡，Huang La)Moxibustion

Melt the wax with fire and drip it onto the skin of the diseased area. It is often used to treat wind-cold-dampness arthralgia, innominate inflammatory swelling, carbuncle, furuncle and eczyma.

3. Burning Rush Moxibustion

Burning rush moxibustion, also called lampwick moxibustion, is performed by applying a burning oiled rush directly on an acupoint and then immediately moving it away. This method is usually employed for children. *Compendium of Material Medica*(本草纲目，Ben Cao Gang Mu) says, "Burning rush moxibustion can be used to treat spasm, coma, clonic convulsion, superduction in children and swelling pain of the head due to wind. A burning oiled rush should be applied on Taiyang(EX-HN5). This method can also be used to relieve the swelling pain due to external hemorrhoids. " *Secrets for Children's Wind-Syndrom of the Head*(小儿惊风秘诀，Xiao Er Jing Feng Mi Jue) says, "Convulsion in children can be treated by applying burning rush moxibustion over the fontanel or between the eyebrow; for superduction, around the umbilicus; for unconsciousness, around the centers of palms and soles; for fixed fist and blank staring, around the center of the vertex; for lockjaw, around the mouth and the centers of palms and soles. "

A Collection of Pediatrics(幼幼集成，You You Ji Cheng) speaks highly of this type of moxibustion and regards it as the first choice for pediatrics. Its function is to dispel wind, relieve exterior syndrome, promote circulation of Qi, remove phlegm, relieve stagnation in the chest, restore consciousness and stop clonic convulsions.

Appendix 1   Moxibustions with Other Materials and Their Functions and Indications

The most commonly used moxibustion often uses fire and moxa to treat diseases. Sometimes, other materials can also be used for moxibustion. The followings are the materals that are usually applied in the clinic, of which, some can cause blisters. Therefore, they can also be used as the materials for crude herb moxibustion as well.

(1) Fresh Ginger(生姜,Sheng Jiang)

Fresh ginger can be used for both indirect moxibustion and external application moxibustion. Fresh ginger, with an acrid taste and warm nature, can warm Yang and dispel cold evil. Therefore, it can be used to treat all cold-deficiency syndromes such as vomiting, diarrhea, abdominal pain, emission, impotence, premature ejaculation, sterility, dysmenorrhea, facial paralysis, and arthralgia due to wind-cold-dampness. Fresh ginger can also be applied directly on the area to treat frostbite.

(2) Garlic(大蒜,Da Suan)

Garlic can be used for partition-moxibustion and also for external application moxibustion after it is pounded into a paste. Garlic, with an acrid taste and strong stimulation, can relieve swelling, remove toxic substance, reduce pain and expel evils. It is effective for treating carbuncle, cellulitis, furuncle, snakebite, mass in the abdomen and tuberculosis. Apply the garlic paste on Yongquan(KI 1), hemoptysis and epistaxis can be treated; on Hegu(LI 4), tonsillitis can be treated; and on Yuji(LU 10), inflammation of the throat can be treated.

(3) Monkshood(附子,Fu Zi)

It may be cut into slices or made into mondshood cake and used for partition-moxibustion. Powders of monkshood can also be mixed with vinegar and applied externally. Monkshood, with an acrid taste and extreme hot nature, can warm the kidney and strengthen Yang. Therefore, it can be used to treat all Yang-deficiency syndromes such as impotence, premature ejaculation, emission, aversion to cold, aching pain and a cold feeling in the waist and chronic unhealing ulcer. When the paste of raw monkshood is applied on Yongquan(KI 1), it can treat toothache.

(4) Chinese Green Onion (葱白,Cong Bai)

Onion can be used for partition-moxibustion after it is cut into slices or mashed into paste or external application moxibustion after it is mashed into paste. Chinese green onion, pungent in flavor and warm in property, can expel evils, promote the circulation of Qi, relieve swelling and remove toxic substances; thus it can be used to treat abdominal pain, enuresis, prostitis, hernia and mastitis.

(5) Salt(盐,Yan)

Fill the umbilicus with salt for partition moxibustion. Salt, with salty flavor and cold property, mainly attributes to the Kidney and Stomach Meridians. Salt-partition moxibustion can recuperate the depleted Yang to cure prostration syndromes. In the clinic, it is often used to treat acute abdominal pain, vomiting, diarrhea, dysentery, and prostration syndrome. If the umbilicus is filled with heated fine salt and then a small bag of heated wheat bran, which is mixed with an appropriate amount of vinegar, and is placed on the salt for moxibustion, coma can be treated.

(6) Croton Seed (巴豆,Ba Dou)

An herbal cake, which is made of a mixture of the powder of Croton seed and flour or proper amount of the powder of Coptis root(黄连, Huang Lian), can be used as a material for partition moxibustion. If the non-fat powder of Croton seed and powder of Realgar (雄黄, Xiong Huang) are applied on the mastoid process of the both ears, malaria can be treated. Croton seed, with acrid flavor, hot property and being poisonous, can warm and dredge the meridians, detoxicate and cure sores. In the clinic, Croton seed-partition moxibustion is often used to treat indigestion, abdominal pain, diarrhea, chest pain, and oliguria.

(7) White Pepper(白胡椒, Bai Hu Jiao)

White Pepper-cake can be used for partition moxibustion and external application moxibustion after it is ground into powder. White Pepper, with an acrid taste and a hot property, can warm and disperse cold evil, promote the circulation of Qi and relieve pain. This method can be used to treat arthralgia due to wind-cold-dampness and numbness. By applying the powder on Dazhui(Du 14), malaria can be treated.

(8) Tuber Onion(韭菜, Jiu Cai)

Tuber Onion, with an acrid taste and a warm property, can be used to treat carbuncle and ulcers when they are pounded into a paste for partition-moxibustion.

(9)Rhizo me of Giant Typhonium (白附子, Bai Fu Zi)

Ground into powder, made into the cake and placed on the umbilicus for partition moxibustion, it can be used to treat hernia.

(10) White Mustard Seed(白芥子, Bai Jie Zi)

Ground into powder, mixed with vinegar and applied on the acupoint for moxibustion, white mustard seed, with an acrid taste and warm property, can remove swelling and disperse accumulated evil. Congestion and blistering may occur after application. This method is effective for arthralgia due to wind-cold-dampness, tuberculosis and facial paralysis.

(11) Herbaseu Radix Panunculi(毛茛, Mao Lang)

Mash the fresh leaves into paste and apply it on the acupoint or diseased area. In the beginning, there is heat sensation in the local area. Then the skin turns red, congestive and blisters occur. After blistering, there may appear local pigmentation, but it will disappear by itself. Apply it on Jingqu(LU 8) or Neiguan(PC 6), Dazhui(Du 4), malaria can be treated. Apply it on local areas, cold arthralgia can be treated. Apply it on Hegu(LI 4) and Shaoshang(LU 11) together with salt, acute conjunctivitis can be treated.

(12) Arisarma Tuber (天南星, Tian Nan Xing)

Ground into powder, mixed with the ginger juice and applied on Jiache(ST 2) and Quanliao (SI 18), it can treat facial paralysis.

(13) Schizonepeta Spike(荆芥穗, Jing Jie Sui)

Break the herb into pieces, heat it by frying and put it in a bag for moxibustion. It can treat urticaria.

(14) Common Fenel Fruit(小茴香, Xiao Hui Xiang)

Common Fenel Fruit, with an acrid taste and hot nature, can regulate flow of Qi, dispel cold evil and stop pain. Grind 100g of Common Fenel Fruit into powder, heat it together with 50g of dried ginger powder and 500g of vinegar and apply it to the acupoint or diseased area. Pain in the stomach and abdomen due to cold evil and cold arthralgia can be treated.

(15) Evodia Fruit Fructus Evodiae(吴茱萸, Wu Zhu Yu)

Evodia fruit Fructus Evodiae, with an acrid taste and hot nature, can dispel cold evil and stop pain by ensuring proper downward flow of Qi and fire. Apply the herbal powder which is mixed with vinegar on Yongquan(KI 1), it treats hypertension, aphthous stomatitis and edema in children. When it is combined with Coptis root(Huang lian, 黄连), acute tonsillitis can be treated.

The following materials can also be used for indirect moxibustion:

Pericarpium Zanthoxyli(川椒, Chuan Jiao) moxibustion——for pain due to pyogenic infections, abdominal distention, traumatic injury.

Flour-cake(面饼, Mian Bing) moxibustion——for malignant boils.

Holotrichia Diomphalia(蛴螬, Qi Cao) moxibustion——for tetanus, skin and external diseases.

Kansui root(甘遂, Gan Sui) moxibustion——for dysuria.

Lepidium(葶苈, Ting Li) seek-cake moxibustion——for scrofula and hemorrhoids.

Chinese honeylocust spine(皂角, Zao Jiao) moxibustion——for a bite by a snake, mosquito, bee, centipede, scorpion and other insects.

Toad venom(蟾蜍, Chan Chu) moxibustion——for scrofula and furuncle.

Macrostem Onion Leaf(薤叶, Xie Ye) moxibustion——for skin and external diseases.

Pokeberry root-cake(商陆, Shang Lu) moxibustion——for scrofula and stubbon fistula.

Nutgrass Flatsedge Rhizome(香附, Xiang Fu) cake moxibustion——for subcutaneous nodule, scrofula and arthralgia.

Aucklandia root(木香, Mu Xiang)cake moxibustion——for traumatic injury and stagnation of Qi and blood.

Peach leaves(桃叶, Tao Ye) moxibustion——for malaria.

Henbane root(莨菪, Lang Dang) moxibustion——for scrofula.

Areca seek(槟榔, Bing Lang) moxibustion——for fulminant deafness when the moxa cone, combined with the musk(麝香, She Xiang), is put into external auditory canal.

Radix Ipomoeae(土瓜根, Tu Gua Gen) moxibustion—— for deafness, tinnitus when the moxa cone is put into the external auditory canal.

Earthwarm faeces(蚯蚓泥, Qin Yin Ni) moxibustion—— for scrofula and furuncle when the earthwarm faeces are used as the partition for moxibustion.

Ephedra(麻黄, Ma Huang) moxibustion—— for wind-cold type of common cold, rhinitis and asthma.

Root of Paniculate swallowwort (徐长卿, Xu Chang Qing) moxibustion——for traumatic injury, wind-dampness type of arthralgia, urticaria and rhinallergosis.

Tangerine peel(陈皮, Chen Pi) moxibustion——for stomach and abdominal distention, poor appetite, vomiting and hiccup.

Astor seek(蓖麻仁, Bi Ma Ren) moxibustion——for gatroptosis, hysteroptosis, proctoptosis when moxibustion is done on Baihui(Du 20); and for facial paralysis when moxibustion is done on Yentang(EX—HN3), Xiaguan(ST 7), Yangbai(GB 14)and Jiache(ST 6).

Appendix 2   Cupping

Cupping, also called horn cupping in ancient times, is a method of applying a cup in which a partial vacuum is created on the skin for therapeutic purpose. Pottery cups, bamboo cups, bronze cups and glass cups are all used today. The shape of the cups and the air-vacuuming methods have been greatly improved from glass cupping which draws the air out by fire to liquid cupping which draws the air by negative pressure of boiling water and to air-extracted cupping. There are single cupping, multiple cupping in alignment, quick cupping, blood-letting puncturing cupping and needle-retention cupping.

Cupping has become an important method in treating diseases since it can enlarge the applications and improve the therapeutic effects. The classification of cupping is presented below: (See Fig. 5—10)

1) The Classification of Cups

(1) Bamboo Cup

The bamboo cup is a section of a bamboo shoot, which is 6—9cm in length, 3—6cm in diameter and 0.5—1cm in thickness with one end closed. Make the edge of the cup smooth before using it. Bamboo cups are light, cheap, and durable. Since bamboo is distributed all over China, it is easy to make bamboo cups.

(2) Pottery Cup

The pottery cup is made of pottery clay. It is large in the middle and small at the two ends. Small cups are short and large cups are long. Strong suction is the feature of this type of cups.

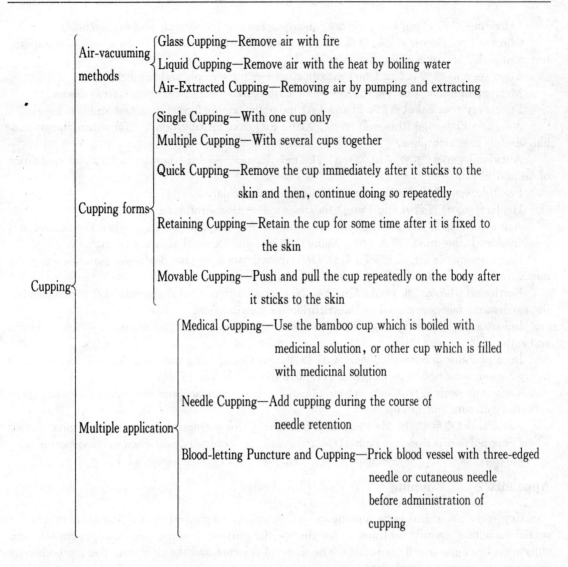

Fig. 5—10   **Classification of Cupping**

(3) Glass Cup

The glass cup comes in different sizes of the large, medium and small type. They are transparent and covenenient for the clinician to observe the condition of congestion and bleeding of the skin and determine the retaining time of the cupping. Glass cups are the ones commonly used today, especially for blood-letting puncturing and needle-retention cupping. (See Fig. 5—11)

2) Cupping Manipulation

(1) Fire Cupping

This method applies negative pressure created by introducing heat in the form of an ignited material to create a vacuum. This causes a jar or cup to be attached to the skin. The manipulations include the following:

A. Fire-Throwing Method

Place a piece of ignited paper into the cup to create a vacuum and immediately place the

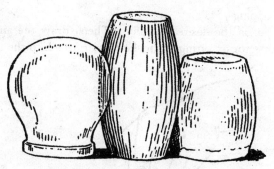

Glass Jar.   Bamboo Jar. Pottery Jar

Fig. 5—11   Type of Jars

mouth of the cup firmly against the skin at the desired location, making the cup or jar attach to the skin. This method is applied only when the cup is required to be attached horizontally. Otherwise, the burning paper may fall and hurt the skin. (See Fig. 5—12)

B. Fire-Twinking Method

Clamp an alcohol cotton ball with the forceps, ignite it and place it into the cup or jar. Then, immediately take it out and place the cup or jar on the selected point or area. Generally the cup or jar may be safely attached to the skin. (See Fig. 5—13)

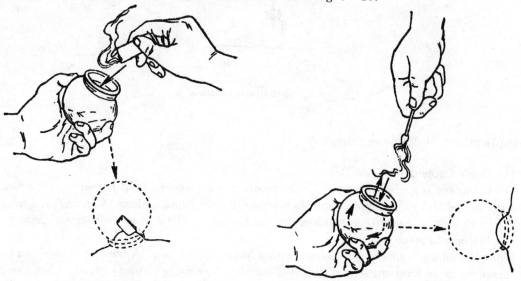

Fig. 5—12   Fire-Throwing Method   **Fig. 5—13   Fire-Twinkling Method**

C. Cotton-Attaching Method

Ignite the alcohol-wetted cotton ball which has been attached to the bottom of the internal wall of the cup and immediately place the cup or jar to the selected point.

D. Material-Placing Method

Place something that is not flammable, heat-resistant and 2—3cm in diameter between the skin and the alcohol cotton ball. Ignite the cotton ball and immediately place the cup or jar on the skin, for a strong suction.

(2) Liquid Cupping

Generally, bamboo cups are applied in this kind of cupping. First boil the cup or jar in a pot. Then take it out, remove the water and immediately attach it to the skin.

(3) Air-Extracted Cupping

Press the aspirating jar on the desired location. Then, draw the air from the cup through the rubber cork with an injector or syringe to make the jar attach to the skin with negative pressure. (See Fig. 5—14)

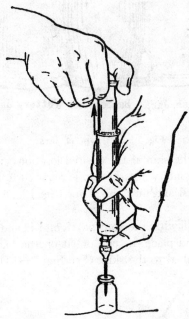

Fig. 5—14   Air-Extracted Method

3) Applications of Various Cuppings

(1) Single Cupping

Single cupping is applied to a small area or painful point. Choose a proper sized cup according to the size of the area to be cupped, and then administer the cupping there. Cupping on Jianyu (LI 15)can be used to treat frozen shoulder and on Zhongwan(RN 12) to treat stomachache.

(2) Multiple Cupping

Multiple cupping is applied for diseases with a large affected area. A number of cups can be used according to the local anatomy of the diseased part. The usage of many cups in a line along a pulled muscle is called multiple cupping in alignment. To treat congestive organs, cups can be fixed on the corresponding area according to the internal anatomy.

(3) Quick Cupping

Place a jar or cup sucked on the skin with the fire-twinking method and then immediately remove it. Repeat this procedure many times until the skin turns red. This method is used for local numbness or hypofunction of the body due to deficiency.

(4) Retaining Cupping

Retain the cup for 5—15 minutes after it is sucked on the skin. The retaining time can be appropriately cut down when a large cup is used with strong suction,or when cupping is conducted on thin muscle areas, or during summer.

(5) Moving Cupping

Moving cupping, also termed pushing cupping, is applied to a large area with abundant muscles such as the loin, back and thigh. Select large glass cups and spread a little oil around the edge of the cups before cupping. After the cup is sucked on the skin, hold the jar or cup with the right hand, move the cup slowly with the back rim pressed and the front rim slightly lifted. Repeat the course several times until the skin turns red. (See Fig. 5—15)

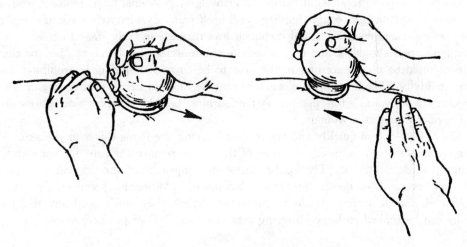

Fig. 5—15　Moving Cupping

(6) Drug Cupping

Make a prescription with Chinese herbal drugs, boil the drugs with water to the proper consistency, and then put the bamboo jar into the fluid to boil again for about 15 minutes. Take the jar out with forceps, eliminate the fluid in the jar and press the hot jar over the selected area. The jar will be sucked to the skin spontaneously. This method is usually used to treat painful syndromes due to wind-dampness. The commonly-used drugs in the prescription are as follows:

Chinese ephedra(麻黄,Ma Huang)6g

Moxa(蕲艾,Qi Ai)6g

Rhizome or root of Notopterygium(羌活,Qiang Huo)6g

Angelica(独活,Du Huo)6g

Ledebouriella Root(防风,Fang Feng)6g

Large-leaff Gentian Root(秦艽,Qin Jiao)6g

Chaenimeles Fruit(木瓜,Mu Gua)6g

Pericarpium Zanthoxyli(川椒,Chuan Jiao)6g

Sichuan Aconite Root(乌头,Wu Tou)6g

Stramonium Blossom(蔓陀罗花,Man Tuo Lou Hua)6g

Artwmisia anomala s. Moor(刘寄奴,Liu Ji Nu)6g

Olibanum(乳香,Ru Xiang)6g

Myrrha(没药,Mo Yao)6g

(7) Needle Cupping

Insert a filiform needle into a selected acupoint to induce a needling sensation and retain the needle there. Then, quickly place a jar or cup over the skin where the needle is retained, the needle being inside the jar.

(8) Blood-Letting Puncture and Cupping

After pricking the selected acupoint or area with a sterilized three-edged needle, or other sharp objects according to the different region and requirements, immediately apply cupping there to cause bleeding. This method can strengthen the effect of blood-letting puncturing therapy and is applicable for acute or chronic soft tissue injury, neurodermatitis, erysipelas, neuroasthenia and digestive sycosomatic disorders.

4) **Indications and Precautions of Cupping**

Cupping can be used to treat wind-dampness arthralgia, abdominal pain, stomachache, indigestion, headache, common cold, cough, lumbago and back pain, dysmenorrhea, conjunctival congestion and swelling pain, snakebite, and carbuncle and furuncle in early stage.

The cupping areas should be the regions where the muscles are abundant. Jars or cups in different sizes should be used according to the area to be cupped. Cupping is prohibited in the case of skin sensitivity. The areas with ulcer, thin muscles, excess hairs, prominence or depression of the joint are not suitable for cupping. Attention must be paid when cupping is done on the lumbosacral region of pregnant woman.

Ignite the alcohol-cotton quickly and try to avoid having the flame fall onto the skin. After 10-15 minutes, press the muscle beside the edge of the cup to remove the cup. Do not simply lift the fixed cup upward or rotate it. The local redness and congestion of the skin can disappear of themselves after several days. Before the redness disappears, additional cupping on the same region is prohibited. Small blisters should be protected though they don't need any treatment. Gentian violet can be applied on large blistering area after the fluid or pus is drained.

Chapter Six

Micro-Acupuncture Therapy
(Local Acupuncture Therapy)

Micro-acupuncture therapy is also called local acupuncture therapy. According to holographic theory, it is recognized that general body information is reflected in the different micro regions and organs. Each micro-region or organ is representative of each and every part of the body and each representative part will reflect physiological and pathological aspects of its corresponding organ or part. This theory is in keeping with the Traditional Chinese Medicine theory: " the internal organs are expressed in the external body. " Micro-acupuncture therapy is a method for treating diseases by puncturing a representative micro-area of the body to treat the greater whole.

Auricular acupuncture is a representative kind of micro-acupuncture therapy. Since 1950, auricular puncture has gained acknowledgement and has become commonly used. In the past twenty to thirty years, new micro-acupuncture therapies have been developed and there have appeared such therapies as puncturing the scalp, occular or facial areas, nasal and mouth regions, tongue, philtrum, wrist, ankle, hand, foot and the radial side of the second metacarpal bone. Also, other puncturings at the palm of the hand, the sole of the foot, the points of Jiaji, back-shu and abdomine and the finger-pressing at the chest points are also considered to be micro-acupuncture. In this chapter, seven main micro-acupuncture therapies will be introduced.

I. Auricular Acupuncture

Auricular acupuncture refers to the use of filiform needles or other methods to stimulate the auricular points to prevent and treat diseases.

All parts of the human body are represented in the ear and can be used for supplementary diagnosis by inspection, palpation and detection for prevention or treatment of diseases. Both ancient and modern texts have recorded the relationship of the ear with many aspects of body diseases. In recent years auricular acupuncture has been enhanced by combining the experience of ancient and modern clinical practice with experimental research.

1. The Auricule and the Auricular Points

1) The Relationship of the Ear with the Zang-Fu Organs and Meridian-Collateral System

(1) The Relationship between the Ear and the Zang-Fu Organs

In Traditional Chinese Medicine theory, the human body is composed of various systems such as the Zang and Fu organs, the five sense organs, the nine orifices, and the four limbs which are all interdependent of each other. The ear is not only the auditory organ, but also has a close relationship with the Zang and Fu organs. In the book *Plain Questions*(素问, Su Wen) it is stated, "In the theory of the five elements, the south belongs to red in colour and connects with the heart, it is open to the orifice of the ear and stores essence in the heart. The patient with liver disease··· if deficiency type···, deafness···; the Qi is upsurging, leading to headache. Spleen···functional disorder leads to obstruction of the nine orifices. " The book *Classic of Medical Problems* (难经, Nan Jing) also says, "Lung is responsible for the voice and can make the ear hear the voice. "The *Miraculous Pivot*(灵枢, Ling Shu) book states, "Kidney Qi connects with the ear, if the kidney function is normal, the ear can hear the five sounds. "According to the records of the *Internal Classic* (内经, Nei Jing) and *Classic of Medical Problems*(难经, Nan Jing), the physiological function of the ear has a relationship with the heart, liver, spleen, lung and kidney.

In later books, the relationship between the ear and the Zang and Fu organs was discussed in more detail. For example, in the Tang Dynasty, the physician Sun Simiao wrote the book *Thousand Golden Prescriptions*(千金要方, Qian Jin Yao Fang)in which he stated, "The heart is responsible for vitality and the tongue is the orifice of the heart, so the heart Qi is connected to the tongue. If the tongue function is normal, it can distinguish the five flavors. The heart also has a relation with the ear···the heart Qi connects with the tongue which opens the orifice to the ear. " The book *Standards of Diagnosis and Treatment*(证治准绳, Zheng Zhi Zhun Sheng) also says, " Tongue is the heart orifice, but it is not a real orifice. So the heart, as a guest, shares the orifice of the ear with the kidney. " In conclusion, the ear has a close physiological relationship with the Zang and Fu organs. Ancient doctors said, " The internal organs are bound to be reflected in the exterior of the body. " This summarizes the law of the interrelationship of the viscera and surface of the body. The auricle is part of the body surface and it reflects the pathological condition of the internal organs. In many ancient books, it was recorded that ancient doctors observed the shape and color of the auricle to aid in the diagnosis of pathological conditions of the Zang and Fu organs, which further indicates the close relationship of the ear with the Zang-Fu organs.

(2) The Relationship between the Ear and the Meridian and Collateral

The ear has its own collateral. Two thousand and one hundred years ago, the book copied on Silk *Yin-Yang Eleven Meridians*(帛书. 阴阳十一脉经, Bo Shu. Yin Yang Shi Yi Mai Jue Jing) mentioned "the ear meridian" which connected with the upper limbs, eyes, cheek and throat. By the time of the publication of *Internal Classic*(内经, Nei Jing), the ancients had not only referred to the "ear meridian" as the Sanjiao Meridian of the Hand Shaoyang, but they also identified the relationship of the ear with the different twelve meridians, divergents and the muscle regions. For example, the *Miraculous Pivot*(灵枢, Ling Shu) says, "The twelve meridians with the three hundred sixty-five collaterals bring Qi and blood upward to the face and then run through the upper orifices. Its Yang Qi arrives at the eyes, so that one can see, and its Qi arrives at the ear, so that one can hear. "

In the course of circulation, some meridian routes pass directly through the ear. For example, the book *Miraculous Pivot* (灵枢, Ling Shu) states, "The Small Intestine Meridian of the Hand Taiyang has one branch ··· that goes to the ear. The Sanjiao Meridian of the Hand Shaoyang···has one branch···that arises from behind the ear, enters the ear and then proceeds to the anterior part of the ear. The divergent channel of the Large Intestine Meridian of the Hand Yangming enters the ear and meets the other meridians. "There are some meridians which are routed around the ear. For example, *Miraculous Pivot* (灵枢, Ling Shu) says, "The Stomach Meridian of the Foot Yangming···passes anteriorly to the ear. One branch of the Bladder Meridian of the Foot Taiyang··· is routed from the top of the head to the upper angle of the auricle. " *Miraculous Pivot* (灵枢, Ling Shu) also mentions that the ear has a relationship with muscle regions of Foot Yangming, Foot Shaoyang and Hand Shaoyang. According to the *Miraculous Pivot* (灵枢, Ling Shu), the three Hand Yang and three Foot Yang Meridians are closely related with the auricular region. Though the six Yin meridians do not directly enter the ear, they meet with the six Yang meridians through their divergent channels. Therefore, all the twelve meridians directly or indirectly enter the ear. So *Miraculous Pivot* (灵枢, Ling Shu) says that all the meridians connect at the ear. As we can see, the ear's relationship with the body is well indicated. When one punctures an auricular point, the sensation will follow a meridian route. If one punctures the twelve Jing-(Well)point, sensation can arrive at the ear. Some patients may be able to feel eight meridian sensations arriving at the ear. At this time, research is being conducted to verify these facts.

2) **Anatomical Structure of the Auricule**

(1) Anatomical Terminology of the Anterior Aspect of the Auricular Surface (See Fig. 6—1)

Helix: The curling rim of the lateral border of the auricle.

Helix Tubercle: A small tubercle at the postero-superior aspect of the helix.

Helix Cauda: The inferior part of the helix, at the junction of the helix and lobule.

Helix Crus: A part of the helix which transverses the auricular cavity.

Antihelix: At the medial aspect of the helix, an elevated ridge parallel to the helix.

Superior Antihelix Crus: The superior of the two branches of the antihelix.

Inferior Antihelix Crus: The inferior of the two branches of the antihelix.

Triangular Fossa: The triangular depression between the two crus of the antihelix.

Scapha: The depression between the helix and the antihelix.

Tragus: A curved flap in front of the auricle.

Supratragic Notch: The concave part between the upper border of the tragus and helix crus.

Antitragus: A small projecting part of the lower part of the antihelix, opposite to the tragus and superior to the ear lobe, curving anteriorly.

Intertragic Notch: the depression between the tragus and antitragus.

Notch between Antitragus and Antihelix: The small depression between the antitragus and antihelix.

Cymba Conchae: The cavity superior to the helix crus.

Cavum Conchae: The cavity inferior to the helix crus.

Orifice of the External Auditory Meatus: The orifice lying in the cavity of the conchae and covered by the tragus.

Ear Lobe: The lowest part of the auricle where there is no cartilage.

(2) Anatomical Terminology of the Posterior Aspect of the Auricular Surface.

Back of Helix: Lateral aspect of the helix where the curling rim is forward.

Back of Helix Cauda: Plane part between the backs of the elevated ridge of the scapha and ear lobe.

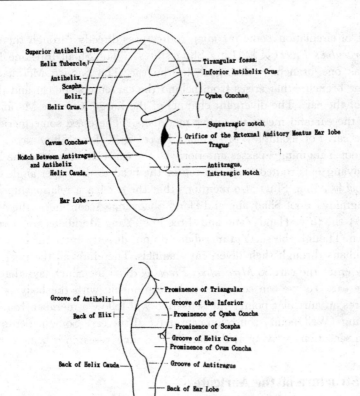

Fig. 6－1 The Anatomical Structure of the Auricular Surface

Back of Ear Lobe：Plaine part of the back of the ear lobe.

Groove of Antihelix：Depression between the backs of the Superior Antihelix Crus and principal part of the helix.

Groove of the Inferior Antihelix Crus：Back of the inferior antihelix crus, a depression from medio-superior close to the latero-inferior aspect.

Groove of Helix Crus：Back of the helix crus which is divided into two branches towards the medio-superior aspect. This is an unclear structure in most people.

Groove of Antitragus：Back depression of the antitragus prominence.

Prominence of Scapha：Back part of the scapha.

Prominence of Triangular Fossa：Back aspect of the triangular fossa in the depression between the two crura of the antihelix.

Prominence of Cymba Concha：Back prominence of cymba concha.

3) Distribution of the Auricular Points

There is a certain regularity in the distribution of the auricular points. These points resemble a fetus with the head downwards, the gluteal region and lower limbs upwards; and the chest, abdomen and trunk in the middle. Generally speaking, points located on the lobule are related to the head and facial region, those on the scapha to the upper limbs, those on the antihelix and its two crura to the trunk and lower limbs, and those in the cavum and cumba conchae to the internal organs. The auricular points are located as follows：

(1) Point(Pt.)Middle Ear is located on the helix crus. The distribution of the auricular points on the helix are Pt. Rectum, Pt. Urethra, Pt. External Genitalia, Pt. Front Ear Apex, Pt. Ear Apex, Pt. Ear tubercle and Pt. Helix 1－6.

(2) The points related to the upper limbs are located on the scapha.

(3) The points related to the trunk and lower limbs are located on the medial border of anti-helix and Point(Pt.)Spinal Column is located on the medial border of antihelix.

(4) Point(Pt.)External Ear and Pt. External Nose are located on the lateral aspect of the tragus; Pt. Supratragic Apex and Pt. Infratragic Apex are on the border of the tragus and Pt. Pharynx-Larynx and Pt. Internal Nose are on the medial aspect of the tragus.

(5)Point(Pt.)Occiput, Pt. Temple and Pt. Forehead are located on the lateral aspect of the antitragus, Pt. Antitragic Apex is on the tip of the antitragus; Pt. Middle border is on the middle between the antitragus apex and Intertragic notch and Pt. Brain and Pt. Subcortex are on the medial aspect of the antitragus.

(6)Point(Pt.)Ear-shenmen, Pt. Pelivic Cavity, Pt. Internal Genitalia and Pt. Superior Fossa are located on the triangular fossa.

(7) The points related to the internal organs are located on the cavum and cymba conchae, of which the points related to the digestive tract are arranged around the helix crus as follows:Pt. Mouth, Pt. Esophagus, Pt. Cardisc Orifice, Pt. Stomach, Pt. Duodenum, Pt. Small Intestine, Pt. Appendix and Pt. large Intestine. Pt. Stomach is around the area where the helix crus termi-nates. Pt. Liver is located at the posterior aspect of the Pt. Stomach and Pt. Duodenum. Pt. Kid-ney is directly above Pt. Small Intestine. Pt. Bladder is directly above Pt. Large Intestine. Pt. Pancreas-Biliary tract is located between the Pt. Liver and Pt. Kidney. Pt. Spleen is located at the inferior aspect of Pt. Liver, close to the border of the antihelix. Pt. Heart is in the center of the central depression of the cavum conchae. The area which resembles the shape of a hoof at the an-terior, posterior and inferior aspects of the Pt. Heart is the lung region, where Pt. Trachae is lo-cated between Pt. Heart and Pt. Mouth. Pt. Sanjiao is located among the Pt. mouth, Pt. En-docrine, Pt. Subcortex and the Lung region.

(8) Point(Pt.)Eye is located at the center of the ear lobe. Pt. Tooth is located antero-superi-or to Pt. Eye. Pt. Tongue is superoir to Pt. Eye. Pt. Jaw is postero-superior to Pt. Eye. Pt. Ante-rior of Ear Lobe is at the anterior aspect, Pt. Internal Ear is at the posterior aspect and Pt. Tonsil is at the directly inferior.

(9) The points on the back of the auricle are Pt. Superior Root of Auricle, Pt. Middle Por-tion of Auricle, Inferior Root of Auricle, Pt. Groove of the Back of the Auricle as well as the points of Heart, Liver, Spleen, Lung and kidney.

4) Location and Indications of Commonly used Ear Points

There are 93 commonly used ear points on the auricula. (See Fig. 6－2) The location and in-dications of the points are introduced as follows. (See Tab. 6－1)

5) Diagnostic Method of Auricular Points

When the human body is ill, a corresponding area in the auricle will reflect it. For example, liver diseases will cause a reaction in the liver area of the ear. Likewise, kidney diseases will cause a reaction in the kidney area. Stimulating the reflective will provide a good result on the affected organ. However, as the shape, size and distribution of auricular areas vary with patients, the re-flective areas also vary. In the clinic, the practitioner should not be limited to the locations and re-active areas marked on the auricular point figure or model, but should examine the patient care-fully and make a diagnosis based on the differentiation of syndromes to determine the root of the disease.

In the clinic, the commonly used diagnosis methods are as follows:

(1) Inspection Method

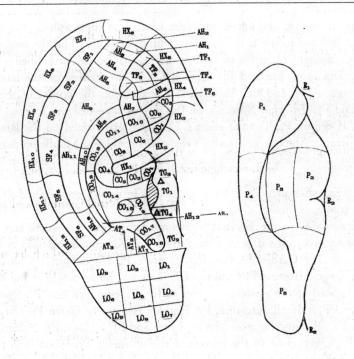

HX$_1$ Ear Center   HX$_2$ Rectum   HX$_3$ Urethra   HX$_4$ external Genitals
HX$_5$ Anus   HX$_{6,7}$ Ear Apes   HX$_8$ Node   Helix 1
HX$_{10}$ Helix 2   HX$_{11}$ Helix 3   HX$_{12}$ Helix 4
SF$_1$ FINGER   SF$_2$ Wrist   SF$_3$ Elbow   SF$_{4,5}$ Shlulder
SF$_6$ Clavicle
AH$_1$ Hell   AH$_2$ Toe   AH$_3$ Ankle   AH$_4$ Knee
AH$_5$ Hip   AH$_6$ Sciatic Nerve   AH$_{6a}$ Sympathesis AH$_7$ Gluteus
AH$_8$ Abdomen   AH$_9$ Lumbosacral Vertebrae   AH$_{10}$ Chest
AH$_{11}$ Thoracic Vertebrae   AH$_{12}$ Neck   AH$_{13}$ Cervical Vertebrae
TF$_1$ Superior Triangular Fossa   TF$_2$ Internal Genitals
TF$_3$ Middle Triangular Fossa   TF$_4$ Shenmen   TF$_5$ Pelvis
TG$_1$ Upper Tragus TG$_2$ Lower Tragus   TG$_{1u}$ External Ear TG$_{1p}$ Apex of Tragus
TG$_{1,2i}$ External Nose   TG$_{2p}$ Adrenal Gland
TG$_3$ Pharynx and Larynx   TG$_4$ Internal Nose
TG$_{21}$ Anterior Intertragal Notch
AT$_1$ Forehead   AT$_{11}$ Posterior Intertragal Notch   AT$_2$ Temple
AT$_3$ Occiput   AT$_4$ Subcortex   AT$_{1,2,4i}$ Apex of Antitragus
AT$_{2,3,4i}$ Central Rim   AT$_{3,4i}$ Grain Stem
CO$_1$ Mouth   CO$_2$ Esophagus   CO$_3$ Cardia   CO$_4$ Stomach
CO$_5$ duodenum   CO$_6$ Small Intestine   CO$_7$ Lagre Intestinal
CO$_{6,7i}$ Appendix   CO$_8$ Angle of Superior Concha   CO$_9$ Bladder
CO$_{10}$ Kidney   CO$_{9,10i}$ Ureter   CO$_{11}$ Pancreas and Gallbladder
CO$_{12}$ Liver   CO$_{6,10i}$ Center of Superior Concha   CO$_{13}$ Spleen
CO$_{15}$ Heart   CO$_{16}$ Trachea   CO$_{14}$ Lung   CO$_{17}$ Triple Energy
CO$_{18}$ Endocrine
LO$_1$ Tooth   LO$_2$ Tongue   LO$_3$ Jaw   LO$_4$ Anterior Ear Lobe
LO$_5$ Eye   LO$_6$ Internal Ear   LO$_{5,6i}$ Cheek   LO$_{7,8,9}$ Tonsil
P$_1$ Heart of Posterior Surface   P$_2$ Lung of Posterior Surface
P$_3$ Spleen of Posterior Surface   P$_4$ Liver of Posterior Surface
P$_5$ kindey of Posterior Surface   PS Groove of Posterior Surface
R$_1$ Upper Ear Root R$_2$ Root of Ear Vagus   R$_3$ Lower Earj Root

Fig. 6$-$2   **Distribution of Auricular Points**

Under natural light, either with the naked eye or using magnification, examine any change in ear color or shape from upper to lower and from the interior to the exterior. Observe any blistering, papules, flaking, congestion or pigmentation. Also observe the shape and color of the blood vessels of the ear.

Tab. 6—1   **Location and Indications of Commonly Used Ear Points**

Anatomical Name	Name of Ear Point	Anatomical Location	Indications
Helix Crus and Helix	Inner ear	At the Helix Crus	Hiccup, dermatosis, Some bleeding diseases
	Rectum	On the end of helix approximate to superior tragic notch	Constipation, prolapse of anus, tenesmus
	Urethra	On the helix at level with the lower border of inferior antihelix crus	Enuresis, frequent micturition, retention of urine
	External genitalia	On the helix at level with the upper border of inferior antihelix tragus	Orchitis, vaginitis, impotence
	Anus	At the Helix inferior to the triangular fossa	Referring point for diagnosis hemorrhoid, hemorrhoid
	Ear apex	At the tip of the auricle when the helix is folded toward tragus	Ocular diseases, mumps, fever, hypertention
	Tubercle	At the tubercle of the Helix	Urticaria, wheal
	Helix 1—4	The region from lower border of auricular tubercle to midpoint of lower border of lobule is divided in three equal parts. The points marking tre divisions are respectively Helix 1—4	Fever, upper respiratory infection

Anatomical Name	Name of Ear Point	Anatomical Location	Indications
Scapha	Finger	At the scapha, above the auricular tubercle	Pain at corresponding area of finger
	Wrist	At the scapha, level with auricular tubercle	Pain at corresponding area of wrist
	Fengxi	Between Pt. Finger and Pt. wrist	Antipruritus, antisensitization, urticaria
	Shoulder	At the scapha, lever with Supratragic notch	Periarthritis, stiff neck
	Elbow	Midway between Pt. wrist and Pt. shoulder	Pain at corresponding area of elbow
	Clavicle	Level with notch between antitragus and antihelix, near helix cauda	Pain at correspnding area of clavicle
Superior crus of antihelix	Toe	At superior and lateral angle of superior and antihelix crus	Toe pain, onychia
	Heel	At superior and medial angle of superior and antihelix crus	Pain at corresponding area of heel
	Ankle	Inferior to Pt. Toe and Pt. Heel	Pain at corresponding area of ankle, sprain
	Knee	Where the superior antihelix crus begins, level with superior border of inferior antihelix crus	Pain at corresponding area of Knee, sprain
	Hip	One-third inferior to the superior antihelix crus	Pain at corresponding area of hip, Bi syndrom
Inferior crus of antihelix	Buttocks	At the level 1/3 of the inferior antihelix crus	Sciatica, pain in buttock region
	Sciatic nerve	Anterior 2/3 of the inferior antihelix crus	Sciatica
	Sympathetic	At junction of inferior antihelix crus and medial margin of helix	Spasm and pain in the internal organs

Anatomical Name	Name of Ear Point	Anatomical Location	Indications
Antihelix	Cervical vertebrae	On a curved line of margin of antihelix, near auditory cavity, the lower 1/3	Pain at the corresponding area of the body. stiff neck
	Thoracic vertebrae	The middle 1/3 of the Curved line of margin of antihelix, near auditory cavity	Pain at the corresponding area of the body
	Lumbosacral vertebrae	The upper 1/3 of the curved line of margin of antihelix, near auditory cavity	Pain at the corresponding area of the body
	Neck	At notch between antihelix and antitragus, near scapha	Stiff neck
	Chest	On antihelix, level with supratragic notch	Pain in chest, intercostal neuralgia, mastitis
	Abdomen	On antihelix, level with lower margin of inferior crus of antihelix	Supplementary point for abdominal and pelvic cavity
Triangular Fossa	Ear-Shenmen	At lateral 1/3 of triangular fossa, in the bifurcating point between superior and inferior crura of antihelix	Insomnia, action to ease mind, relieve pain
	Pelvic cavity	Slightly inferior to the medial side of the bifurcating point between the superior and inferior antihelix crus	Pelvic inflammation
	Internal genitalia	In the depression in the midpoint of the bottom of the triangular fossa	Women diseases, impotence
	Superior fossa	Medial superior to the triangular fossa	Hypertention

Anatomical Name	Name of Ear Point	Anatomical Location	Indications
Tragus	External ear	At the depression slightly anterior to the supratragic notch	Tinnitus, deafness
	External nose	At the Center of lateral aspect of tragus	Allergic rhinitis
	Tragic apex	At the tip of prominence at the upper tragus	Toothache, squint
	Adrenal gland	At the tip of prominence at the lower tragus	Elevating blood pressure, antisensitization
	Pharynx and largnx	At upper half of the medial aspect of tragus	Acute and chronic throat inflammation
	Internal nose	At the lower half of medial aspect of tragus below pt. Pharynx-Larynx	Tonsillitis, rhinitis
Antitragus	Antitragic Apex	At the antitragus apex	Asthma, mumps
	Middle Border	Midpoint between the antitragic apex and helix tragic notch	Enuresis, insomnia
	Occiput	At the posterior superior corner of the lateral aspect of the antitragus	Headache, neurasthenia
	Temporal	At the midpoint of the lateral aspect of the antitragus	Headache, migraine
	Forehead	At the anterior inferior corner of the lateral aspect of the antitragus	Headache, dizziness, insomnia
	Brain	Upper 1/2 on the medial aspect of the antitragus	Headache, dizziness
	Subcortex	Lower 1/2 on the medial aspect of the antitragus	Calm spirit, stop pain

Anatomical Name	Name of Ear Point	Anatomical Location	Indications
Periphery Helix Crus	Mouth	Close to the posterior and superior border of the orifice of the external auditory meatus	Stomatitis
	Esophagus	At middle 2/3 of the inferior aspect of the helix crus	Esophagitis
	Cardiac Orifice	At lateral 1/3 of the inferior aspect of the helix crus	Nausea, Vomiting
	Stomach	Around the area where the helix crus terminates	Stomachache, Vomiting, indigestion
	Duodenum	At lateral 1/3 of the superior aspect of the helix crus	Duodenal ulcer, pylorospasm
	Small Intestine	At middle 1/3 of the superior aspect of the helix crus	Indigestion, palpitation
	Large Intestine	At medial 1/3 of the superior aspect of the helix crus	Diarrhea, Constipation
	Appendix	Between pt. Small Intestine and pt. Large Intestine	Acute and simple appendicitis
Cymba Conchae	Liver	On the lateral inferior border of the cymba conchae	Diseases of the eye, hypochondriac pain
	Kidney	On the lower border of the inferior antihelix crus	Lumbago, tinnitus, deafness
	Pancrease and Biliary Tract	Between pt. Liver and pt. Kidney	Indigestion, diseases of the biliary tract
	Bladder	On the anterior inferior border of the inferior antihelix crus	Enuresis, retention of urine
	Ureter	Between Pt. Kidney and Pt. Bladder	Diseases of the ureter
	Angle of Cymba Conchae	At the medial superior angle of cymba conchae	Prostatitis
	Middle of Cymba Conchae	At the centre of cymba conchae	Umbilicus pain

Anatomical Name	Name of Ear Point	Anatomical Location	Indications
The Cavum Conchea	Heart	In the central depression of the Cavum Conchae	Hysteria, palpitation
	Lung	Around the central depression of the Cavum Conchae	Cough, skin diseases
	Trachea	Between the orifice of the external auditory meatus and pt. Heart	Asthma
	Spleen	At the lateral and superior aspect of the Cavum Conchae	Abdominal distention, indigestion
	Intertragus	At the base of the Cavum Conchae in the intertragic notch	Dysmenorrhea, irregular menstruation
	Sanjiao	At the base of the Cavum Conchae, superior to the intertragic notch	Constipation, edema
	Endocrine	At the anterior irferior of the Cavum Conchae in the intertragic notch	Menopause syndrome, dysfunction of endocrine
Ear Lobule	Anterior side of the inter-tragic notch	On the anterior and inferior side of the intertragic notch	Glaucoma, pseudomyopia, style
	Posterior side of the inter-tragic notch	On the posterior and inferior aspect of the intertragic notch	Glaucoma, pseudomyopia, style
	Tooth	On the area from the lower border of the cartilage of the intertragic notch to the lower border of the ear lobe, draw three horizontally lines by which the area is horizontally and equally divided, then draw two vertical lines by which the area is vertically and equally divided, thus the area is divided into equal sections. These sections are numbered from the medial section laterally and from the upper section downward. The first section is pt. Tooth; the 2nd, Pt. Tongue; the 3rd. Pt. Jaw; the 4th, Pt. Anterior of Ear lobe; the 5th, Pt. Eye; the 6th, Pt. Internal Ear. Pt. Cheek is around the border line of the 5th and 6th sections. The 8th section is Pt. Tonsil	Corresponding area of toothache, peridentitis, anesthesia of dental extraction
	Tongue		Diseases of the tongue
	Jaw		Mandibular auticulation inflammation
	Anterior of Ear lobe		Corresponding area of toothache, peridentitis
	Eye		Glaucoma, style, pseudomyopia
	Internal Ear		Tinnutis, deafness
	Cheek		Facial paralysis
	Tonsil		Tonsillitis

Anatomical Name	Name of Ear Point	Anatomical Location	Indications
The Back Auricle	Upper Root of Auricle	At the upper chondral prominence on retroauricle	Stop pain, paralysis diseases
	Root of auricular vagus nerve	At the junction of retroauricle and mastoid, level with helix crus	Headache, stuff nose; biliary ascariasis
	Lower portion of Back of Auricle	At the lower chondral prominence of retroauricle	Relieve pain, paralysis diseases
	Groove of Back Auricle	At the groove on retroauricle, running from the upper to the lower obliquely	Hypertension
	Heart	Upper portion of back auricle	Diseases at corresponding area of heart
	Spleen	Middle portion of back auricle	Diseases at corresponding area of spleen
	Liver	Lateral middle portion of back auricle	Diseases at corresponding area of liver
	Lung	Medial middle portion of back auricle	Diseases at corresponding area of lung
	Kidney	Lower portion of back auricle	Diseases at corresponding area of kidney, lumbago

(2) Palpation Method

Use the thumb and index finger to apply pressure at the various locations of the ear from upper to lower and interior to exterior. Note any positive reaction in areas corresponding to body parts or internal organs. Palpation detects verrucous vegetation, scleroma and hypertrophy of the cartilage.

(3) Detection Method

This is the most commonly used diagnostic method at present. After simple diagnosis, the practitioner uses a detecting probe (a small springy metal probe) or the handle of the filiform needle, applying pressure from the periphery to the center, from the upper ear to the lower and from the exterior to the interior. The pressure is applied to the corresponding auricular area of the disease to find pain or sensative points. When the exploring probe applies pressure at a sensitive point, the patient can indicate the location of discomfort as the practitioner passes over it. According to the point of pain, the corresponding anatomical area can be used to aid in determining physical dysfunction or illness of the Zang-Fu organs. For example, if the ear's liver area is sensitive, the practitioner should consider the possibility of liver disease, occular disease or gallbladder disease. When detecting, the practitioner's hand must be mild, slow and apply evenly distributed pressure. Sometimes, some patient's auricular sensitive points may have deformation or abnormal color of the skin and may be extremely sensitive. These are visual aids for identifying problem areas. If it is difficult to find pressure pain points in some patients, first massage the area concerned, and then find the pain points, or detect them at the reactive area of the other ear. If there is still not a painful point, then choose the auricular points according to the symptoms.

(4) Electric Detecting Method

This is a method using specially-made electrical instruments to detect the changes of electrical resistance, potential and capacity on the areas of auricular skin. The auricular reactive points have a lower electrical resistance and higher electrical conductivity than the surrounding skin. A hand-held transistor can detect the points of non-conductivity During detection, the practitioner holds the exploring pole of the transistor to probe the auricular area and the patient holds the oppositely charged pole to complete the circuit. The hand-held transistor emits high frequency noise or illuminates the low electric resistance when the pole passes over an auricular reaction point. This electric detecting method, compared with the pressure pain method, has the advantages of accuracy and simplicity.

(5) Other Methods

Besides the inspection, palpition, detection, ausculation and earache-analysis methods mentioned above, there are others such as the ear points heat sensitivity method (to check temperature at the various auricular areas), the auricular points impressing method (to use pressure and measure the time the blood takes to return to the different auricular areas), the auricular staining method and the auricular reflection method.

2. Clinical Applications of Auricular Acupuncture

Auricular points are the reactive points located in the ear corresponding to the internal organs, four limbs and trunk. These points can be punctured, or stimulated by other means, to treat diseases corresponding with the Zang and Fu organs. In recent years, auricular acupuncture has become more widely used in treating diseases.

1) Clinical Indications of Auricular Acupuncture

Auricular acupuncture can treat approximately two thousand diseases. It is very effective for acute disease, but it is also helpful for chronic disease. Auricular acupuncture is very effective for the following categories of diseases:

(1) All Types of Pain Diseases

Pain due to traumatic injury, such as muscle sprain, twisted injury of the joints, contusion, puncture, incisionary wounds, fractures and stiff neck; pain of the nervous system such as headache, migraine, trigeminal neuralgia, intercostal pain, herpes zoster and sciatica; pain due to post-operative wounds that damage the five sense organs such as cranial, abdominal or thoraxic operations, operations of the four limbs and post-operative discomfort, sequele pain, headache or lumbago secondary to anesthesia.

(2) All Types of Inflammatary Diseases

Auricular acupuncture can be used to eliminate inflammation and stop pain for inflamatory diseases such as acute conjunctivitis, tympanitis, sore throat, tonsillitis, mumps, bronchitis, enteritis, pelvic inflammation, rheumatic arthritis, facial nerve inflammation and peripheral neuritis.

(3) Some Functional Disorders

Auricular acupuncture has bidirectional function to regulate, relieve or cure functional disorders such as dizziness, arrhythmia, hypertension, hyperhidrosis, intestinal dysfunction, irregular menstruation, neurasthenia, enuresis, hysteria and sexual dysfunction.

(4) Allergies and Development of Allergic Reactions

Auricular acupuncture can eliminate inflammation, desensibilizate allergic reactions and improve the immunitary function to strengthen the body against diseases such as allergic rhinitis, asthma, allergic colitis and urticaria.

(5) Endocrine Metabolic Diseases

Auricular acupuncture can reduce symptoms or reduce the dosage of medicines for simple goiter, hypothyroidism, menopause syndrome and simple obesity.

(6) Some Infectious Diseases

Auricular acupuncture can increase the immune defense function to help the body fight against diseases such as influenza, dysentery, malaria and juvenile plane warts.

(7) All Types of Chronic Diseases

Auricular acupuncture can relieve chronic symptoms from diseases such as lumbago, periarthritis of the shoulder, indigestion and numbness of the four limbs.

In addition to the above diseases, auricular acupuncture can be used for anesthesia (auricular anesthesia) and to help stimulate the mother hormones that effect delivery and produce breast milk. The auricular points are very effective strengthening the immunitary system to prevent common cold, sea or car sickness. These points can also prevent and manage reactions to transfusio and are effective in helping patients to quit addictions including smoking, relieve competitive stress and reduce body weight.

2) **Principles for Selecting Auricular Points**

(1) Selecting Points According to Differentiation of Syndromes

The points are chosen according to the differentiation of the theories of Zang-Fu organs, meridians and collaterals of Traditional Chinese Medicine. For example, for dermatosis, the lung points are selected according to the theory that "The lung is responsible for skin and hair". For bone fractures, the kidney points are selected according to the theory, "The kidney is responsible for the bones".

(2) Selecting Points According to Symptoms and Syndromes

Auricular points are chosen according to the syndromes in Chinese Medicine as well as the pathology and physiology in western medicine. For example, for neurasthenia, the auricular subcortex point is selected; for abnormal menstruation, the auricular endocrine point is selected;

(3) Selecting Points According to Diseases

The points are chosen according to the clinical diagnosis of the disease(s). For example, for liver diseases, the auricular liver point is selected. For eye diseases, Pt. eye 1 and Pt. eye 2 are chosen. For nephritis, the auricular kidney point is selected.

(4) Selecting Points According to Clinical Experience

Points are selected based on the practitioner's clinical experience. For example, the Inner Ear Point can be used to treat diaphragm spasm, but also blood diseases and skin diseases. The stomach point can be used to treat digestive diseases and also diseases of the nervous system. The Er Men(Shenmen) Point can stop pain, tranquilize the mind and calm the spirit. The Er Jian Point, when punctured and blood-let, can diminish inflammation, reduce fever and relieve convulsion.

3) **Manipulations and Procedure**

As a rule, the manipulation of auricular acupuncture is similar to the manipulation of body acupuncture. However, in auricular acupuncture, the practitioner must be exact in point location and skilled at needle insertion. Extra care should be taken in skin preparation and sterilization. Also, attention must be given to the time of needle retention to avoid secondary reactions or infection.

Point selection should be first done according to the diagnosis of the disease which will be referred to later as the prescription. The practitioner must find the sensitive spot or reactive point within the prescription area. If a sensitivity or reactive point is not found, then puncture the points indicated for the disease.

Strict sterilization procedures must be followed for auricular acupuncture because it is easy for the auricular cartilage to get inflamed. The practitioner must observe two aspects of sterilization. The first is the sterilization of the needles, and the second is the sterilization of the skin. For the disinfection, first use 2% iodine tincture, then 75% alcohol to sterilize and deiodinize the skin.

(1) Puncture with the Filiform Needle

Generally the patient is in a sitting position for treatment. However, if the patient is nervous, afraid of pain or constitutionally weak, he or she should lie down. Use sterile stainless steel needles #24 to #30 in diameter and 0.3 to 1.0 cun in length. The #28, 0.5 cun stainless needle is most commonly used.

A. Insertion of the Needle

To insert the needle, the practitioner uses the thumb and index finger of the left hand to secure the ear. The middle finger of the left hand is positioned on the back side of the ear for support to reduce pain while puncturing and aid in the control of the depth of insertion. The practitioner holds the needle with the thumb and index finger of the right hand to insert at a pressure painful point or the indicated point. The needle may be inserted either by the quick or by the slow method.

The quick insertion method requires skilled manipulation with the practitioner using force from the wrist and the finger. Twirl and quickly insert the needle perpendicularly into the auricular cartilage at the pressure pain point. Special care must be taken not to puncture through the cartilage. The patient should inhale deeply through the mouth at the moment of insertion to relieve the pain. Needle insertion should be steady, accurate and quick.

The slow insertion method requires a coordinated slow insertion by twirling the needle with steady and well-distributed force.

There are three types of manipulations commonly used in the clinic.

ⓐMere Insertion Method

Puncture a pressure painful point and retain the needle immediately without any manipulation. This method is used for the senile, constitutionally weak patient, or children.

ⓑTwirling Method

After insertion, use moderate stimulation and twirl the needle clockwise with small amplitude. Continue stimulating by twirling for one to two minutes. This method is used for chronic diseases.

ⓒLifting and Thrusting Method

After perpendicular insertion, lift and thrust the needle to increase stimulation for one to two minutes. This method is used for pain and acute diseases.

B. Depth of Puncture

The puncture depth depends on the thickness of the patients ear. Generally it is 0.2—Z0.3 cun; that is, the needle can be secure in the cartilage of the auricle.

C. Retaining of the Needle

Generally the needle is retained for twenty to thirty minutes. For chronic and painful diseases, the needle may be retained for a longer period. For children and senile patients the time of retention may be shorter. During needle-retenting time, stimulation done every ten mimutes will increase the effect.

D. Withdrawing of the Needle

The practitioner should use the left hand to secure the back of the ear and the right hand to withdraw the needle. There are two methods to withdraw the needle.

ⓐQuickly Withdrawing Method

Quickly and perpendicularly take out the needle. This method can prevent pain.

ⓑTwirling-Withdrawing Method

Just before withdrawal, give a final twirling stimulation and then withdraw the needle. This method is used for patients who haven't experienced a very good effect in treatment.

After withdrawing the needle, use a sterile dry cotton to apply pressure on the hole to avoid bleeding. Clean the puncture hole with iodine tincture.

(2) Electro-Acupuncture

Electric auricular acupuncture combines the application of the filiform needle and stimulation with electric pulsing current. Different patterns of pulse or wave may be used to stimulate the auricular points to increase the effect. Electric acupuncture can be applied to all of the auricular points to treat diseases. It is commonly used for diseases of the nervous system, visceral spasm pain and asthma. Electric auricular acupuncture is extensively used for acupuncture anesthesia.

(3) Puncture by Needle Embedding Method

This is a method to bury the intradermal needle into the auricular cartilage to treat disease. It is used for pain and chronic diseases to provide continuous stimulation to strengthen the curative effect or to avoid recurrances. First, follow all the precautions to sterilize the skin. The practitioner uses the left hand to secure the auricle and the tweezers in the right hand to hold the sterile intradermal needle and lightly insert the needle into the skin. Generally, insert two thirds of the needle body into the cartilage and then fix the needle in place with an adhesive plaster. Usually only puncture the auricle of the affected or diseased side. If the situation of the disease requires both sides, the practitioner may embed needles in both ears. Stimulate the embedded area by having the patient press three times a day and retain the needles for three to five days at a time.

II. Scalp Acupuncture

Scalp acupuncture is a method that can treat diseases of the body by puncturing certain points or by stimulating areas that correspond to the cerebro-cortical distribution functions of the scalp.

1. The Relationship of the Head with the Zang-Fu Organs and Meridian-Collaterals System.

In the book *Plain Quetions*(素问, Su Wen), it was pointed out that, "The head is the residence of the spirit". Later, a physician Zhang Jiebing explained this quotation as "The Qi and vital essence of the five Zang and six Fu organs all ascend to the head". All this indicates the close relationship of the head with the Zang-Fu organs of the body.

The head is the confluential area of the Yang Qi. All the six hand and six foot Yang meridians pass through the head. The hand and foot Yangming Meridians are distributed in the forehead and face. The Stomach Meridian of the Foot Yangming "starts from the lateral side of the ala nasi and ascends to the bridge of the nose where it meets the Bladder Meridian of the Foot Taiyang, then it descends downwards along the lateral side of the nose···, turning to ascend in front of the ear, transversing Shangguan(GB 3), and then following the anterior hairline, finally reach the forehead···". The hand and foot Shaoyang Meridians are distributed in the lateral side of the head. The auricular branch of the Sanjiao Meridian of the Hand Shaoyang "arises from the retroauricular region and enters the ear, crosses a previous branch at the cheek and reaches the outer canthus". The Gallbladder Meridian of the Foot Shaoyang "originates from the outer canthus and ascends to the corner of the forehead where it curves downward to the retroauricular region and runs along the side of the neck in front of the Sanjiao Meridian of the Hand Shaoyang··· the retroauricular branch of this meridian arises from the retroauricular region and enters the ear. Then, it comes out and passes through the preauricular region to the posterior aspect of the outer canthus···"

The hand and foot Taiyang Meridians are distributed in the cheek and neck regions. The Bladder Meridian of the Foot Taiyang starts at the inner canthus, ascends to the forehead and joins the Du Meridian at the vertex, where a branch rises and runs to the temple. The straight portion of the meridian enters and communicates with the brain from the vertex. Then it emerges and bifurcates to descend along the posterior aspect of the neck.

The Du Meridian "runs posteriorly along the interior of the spinal column to Fengfu (DU 16) at the nape, where it enters the brain. Then it further ascends to the vertex and runs along the forehead to the columnella of the nose".

Of the six Yin meridians, only the Pericardium Meridian of the Hand Shaoyin and Liver Meridian of the Foot Jueyin directly pass through the head and face. The Liver Meridian of Foot Jueyin "ascends along the posterior aspect of the throat to the nasal pharynx and connects with the eye system (i. e. the tissues connecting the eyes with the brain.), then runs further upward and emerges from the forehead and meets with the Du Meridian at the vertex. The branch which arises from the eye system runs downward into the cheek and curves around the inner surface of the lips. "

The other Yin meridians indirectly arrive at the head via their divergence with the Yang meridians. Thus, the meridian Qi of the whole body concentrates at the head. T. C. M theory states "the Qi originates from the brain" which indicates that the head is an important confluential area for the Qi of the whole body. Therefore, scalp acupuncture has a good effect and a large spectrum of applications in treatment.

2. Location and Indications of Stimulation Areas on the Scalp

In order to precisely locate the stimulation areas on the scalp, two standard lines have been devised:

The antero-postero medial line——The line connecting the midpoint between the two eyebrows and the midpoint of the lower border of the external occipital protuberance. (See Fig. 6—3)

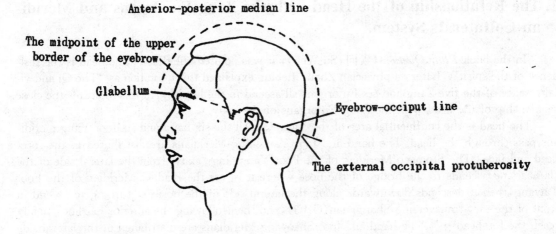

Fig. 6—3 The stimulation Areas on the Scalp (1)

The eyebrow-occiput line——The horizontal line connecting the midpoint of the upper border of the eyebrow and the highest prominence of the external occipital protuberance.

The commonly used stimulation areas on the scalp are as follows:

(1) Motor Area

Location: The motor area is equal to the projection of the precentral gyrus of the cerebral cortex on the scalp. Its upper point is 0. 5cm posterior to the midpoint of the antero-posterior medial line, while its lower point is at the junction of the eyebrow-occipital line and the temporal hair line. The connecting line between these two points is the motor area. The motor area is divided into 5 equal parts: the upper 1/5 is the lower limb and trunk; the middle 2/5 is the upper limbs motor area; and the lower 2/5 is the face motor area (See Fig. 6—4).

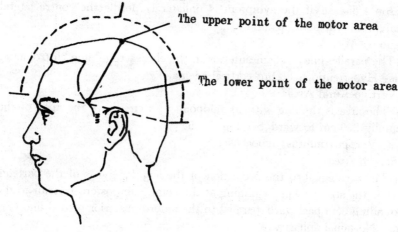

Fig. 6—4　the Stimulation Areas on the Scalp (2)

Indications: The upper 1/5 of the motor area is used for contra-lateral paralysis of the lower limb. The middle 2/5 of the motor area is for contra-lateral paralysis of the upper limb. The lower 2/5 of the motor area is for contra-lateral central facial paralysis, motor aphasia, abnormal salivation or dysphonia.

(2) Sensory Area

Location: The sensory area is equal to the projection of the postcentral gyrus of the cerebral cortex on the scalp. The parallel line, 1.5cm posterior to the motor area, is the sensory area. The upper 1/5 of this area is the lower limbs, head and trunk sensory areas; the middle 2/5 is the upper limb sensory area; and the lower 2/5 is the face sensory area (See Fig. 6—5)

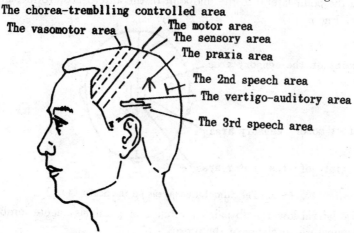

Fig. 6—5　The Stimulation Areas on the Scalp (3)

Indications: The upper 1/5 of the sensory area is for contra-lateral lumbar and leg pain, numbness and paresthesia, headache in the nape region, and tinnitus; the middle 2/5 is for contra-lateral upper limb pain, numbness and paresthesia; and the lower 1/5 is for contra-lateral facial numbness, migraine, trigeminal neuralgia, toothache, and temporo-madibular arthritis.

In the scalp, acupuncture anesthesia is employed in surgical operations on the relevant part of the body. The sensory area is used in combination with the visceral areas (i.e. the thoracic, gastric and reproduction areas).

(3) Chorea-Tremblling Controlled Area

Location: The parallel line, 1.5cm anterior to the motor area (See Fig. 6—5) Indications: Chorea, Parkinson's disease (if the symptom is unilateral, needle the contra-lateral stimulation area; if bilateral, needle the area bilaterally).

(4) Vasomotor Area

Location: The parallel line, 1.5cm anterior to the chorea-trembling cintrol area.

Indications: Hypertention, cerebro-cortical edema.

(5) The Vertigo-Aural Area

Location: The area is the line with its midpoint 1.5 cm above the apex of the auricle, extending horizontally 2.0 cm forward (See Fig. 6—5)

Indications: Vertigo, tinnitus, hypoacusia.

(6) 2nd Speech Area

Location: The area equal to the projection of the angular gyrus of the parietal lobe on the scalp. This area is the straight line beginning at the point 2cm postero-inferior to the parietal tubercle, and extending 3cm backward, parallel to the antero-posterior medial line (See Fig. 6—5)

Indications: Norminal aphasia.

(7) 3rd Speech Area

Location: A horizontal line 4cm backward horizontal line from the midpoint of the vertigo-auditory area (See Fig. 6—5)

Indication: Sensory aphasia.

(8) Praxia Area

Location: The area referring to the three lines beginning from the parietal tubercle. One line extends vertically downward 3cm and the others extend anteriorly and posteriorly 3cm at a 40° angle with the former line respectively (See Fig. 6—5)

Indications: Apraxia.

(9) Foot Motor Sensory Area

Location: The area referring to two straight lines parallel to the anterior-posterior median line, beginning from the point lateral to the midpoint of the antero-postero medial line extending 3cm backward. (See Fig. 6—6)

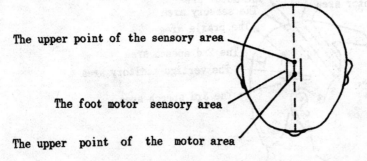

The upper point of the sensory area

The foot motor sensory area

The upper point of the motor area

Fig. 6—6   The Stimulation Areas on the Scalp (4)

Indications: Contral-lateral lower limb pain, numbness or paralysis, acute lumbar sprain, cerebro-cortical polyuria, nocturia, prolapse of the uterus.

(10) Visual Area

Location: The area referring to two straight lines parallel to the antero-posterior medial line beginning from the point 1cm lateral to the external occipital protuberance and extending 4cm upward. (See Fig. 6—7)

Indications: Cerebro-cortical visual disorders.

(11) Balance Area

Location: The area referrings to two straight lines parallel to the antero-postero medial line, beginning from the point 3.5cm lateral to the external occipital protuberance and extending 4cm downward. (See Fig. 6—7)

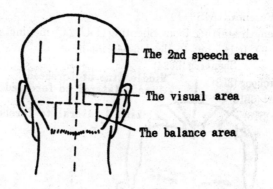

Fig. 6—7   The Stimulation Areas on the Scalp (5)

Indications: Equilibrium disorders caused by cereballum disease.

(12) Stomach Area

Location: The area referring to two lines parallel to the antero-postero medial line, beginning from the cross point of the straight line, ascending vertically from the pupil and the anterior hair line, extending 2cm upward. (See Fig. 6—8)

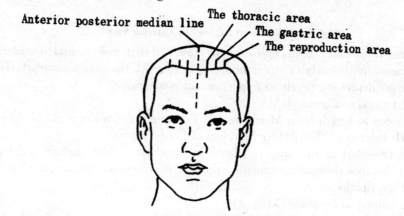

Fig. 6—8   The Stimulation Areas on the Scalp (6)

Indications: Gastric pain, epigastric discomfort.

(13) Thoracic Area

Location: The area referring to two lines, parallel to the antero-postero medial line, between the gastric area and the antero-postero medial line, extending from the anterior hair margin upward 2cm and downward 2cm, (See Fig. 6—8)

Indications: Chest pain and stuffiness, palpitation, coronary heart disease, heart failure, asthma and hiccup.

(14) Reproduction Area

Location: The area referring to a 2cm line parallel to the antero-postero medial line, beginning from the forehead corner extending upward. (See Fig. 6—8)

Indications: Functional uterine bleeding, pelvic inflammation, leukorrhagia. Prolapse of uterus can be treated in association with the foot motor sensory area.

3. Location and Indications of the Standard Nomenclature of Scalp Acupuncture Lines

There are 14 standard nomenclatures of scalp acupuncture lines which are related as follows:

(1) Middle Line of Forehead(MS—1)

Location: 1 cun in length starting from Shenting(DU 24) moving straight down along the Du Meridian(See Fig. 6—9). It belongs to the Du Meridian.

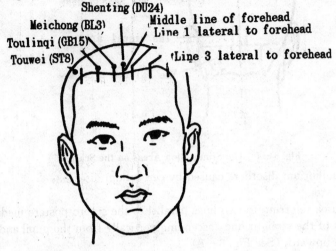

Fig. 6—9 Forehead Region (in Anterior View)

Indications: Diseases of head, nose, tongue, eye, throat and mental disorders such as headache, dizziness, ophthalmalgia, stuffy nose, rigid tougue, tinntus, sorethroat, facial pain, insomnia, amnesia, depressive psychosis, epilepsy and convulsion

(2) Line 1 Lateral to Forehead(MS—2)

Location: 1 cun in length from Meichong(BL 3) straight down along the Bladder Meridian (See Fig. 6—9)It belongs to the Bladder Meridian of Foot-Taiyang.

Indications: Disorders of the lung and heart in upper-jiao which include cough, asthma, chest distress, palpitation, insomnia, amnesia, thoracic obstruction, epigastralgia, aphasia with stiff tongue and angiopathy.

(3) Line 2 Lateral to Forehead(MS—3)

Location: 1 cun in length from Toulinqi(GB 15)straight down along the Gallbladder Meridian(See Fig. 6—9). It belongs to the Gallbladder Meridian of Foot-Taiyang.

Indications: Disorders of the spleen, stomach, liver, gallbladder and pancreas in the middle-jiao such as stomacheache, neasia, vomiting, hiccup, abdominal pain, diarrhea, hypochondrium pain, mammary swelling and pain, vertigo and eye diseases.

(4) Line 3 Lateral to Forehead(MS—4)

Location: 1 cun in length from the point 0.75 cun medial straight downwardsto Touwei (St 8) (See Fig. 6—9). It belongs to the Bladder Meridian of Foot-Taiyang and the Stomach Meridian of Foot-Yangming.

Indications: Disorders of the kidney and urinary bladder in the lower-jiao such as urinary incontineunce, enuresis, impotence, seminal emission and chronic diarrhea as well.

(5) Middle Line of Vertex(MS—5)

Location: From Baihui(DU 20)to Qianding(DU 21)along the Du Meridian 1.5 cun in length)(See Fig. 6—10). It belongs to the Du Meridian.

Indications: Disorders of the waist and lower limbs such as paralysis, numbness and pain; cortical polyuria, prolapse of anus, infantile nocturnal enuresis, dizziness, insomnia, poor memory, headache, epilepsy and other mental disorders.

(6) Anterior Oblique Line of Vertex-Temporal(MS—6)

Location: From Qianshenchong(1 cun anterior to Baihui(DU 20)) obliquely to Xuanli(GB

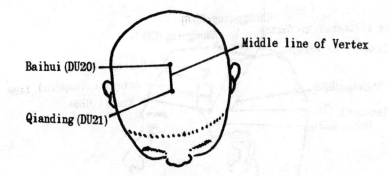

Fig. 6—10   The Puncturing Line on Vertex Region

6), passing across the Du Meridian, the Bladder Meridian of Foot-Taiyang and the Gallbladder Meridian of Foot-Shaoyang(See Fig. 6—11).

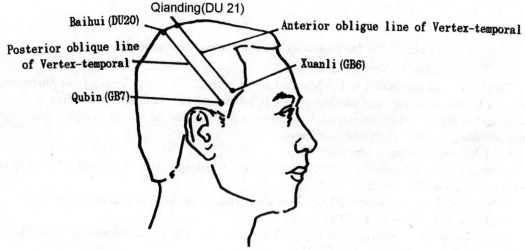

Fig. 6—11   The Puncturing Lines on Vertex-Temporal Region

Indications: The line is divided equally into five portions. The upper 1/5 is indicated in paralysis of contralateral lower limbs; the middle 2/5 in paralysis of contralaternal upper limbs and the lower 2/5 in facial paralysis, motor aphasia, abnormal salivation and cerebral arterioesclerosis. It is mainly for contra-lateral motor functional disorders.

(7) Posterior Oblique Line of Vertex-Temporal(MS—7)

Location: From Baihui(DU 20)obliquely to Qubin(GB 7), passing across the Du Meridian, the Bladder Meridian of Foot-Taiyang and Gallbladder Meridian of Foot-Shaoyang(See Fig. 6—11).

Indications: The line is divided equally into five portions. The upper 1/5 is indicated in pain, numbness and itch of lower limbs; the middle 2/5 in pain, numbness and itch of upper limbs; and the lower 2/5 in pain, numbness and itch of head and face. It is mainly for contra-lateral sensory functional disorders.

(8) Line 1 Lateral to Vertex(MS—8)

Location: 1.5 cun lateral to Middle Line of Vertex, 1.5 cun in length from Chengguang (BL 6)backward along the Foot-Taiyang. It belongs to the Bladder Meridian of Foot-Taiyang (See Fig. 6—12).

Indications: Disorders of the waist and legs such as paralysis, pain, numbness and functional disorders of lower limbs. It is mainly for a contra-lateral motor functional disorder.

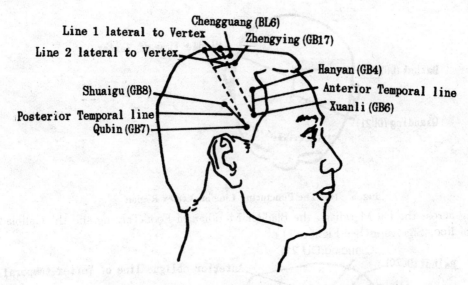

Fig. 6-12 The Puncturing Lines on Vertex-Temporal Region

(9) Line 2 Lateral to Vertex(MS-9)

Location: 2. 25 cun lateral to the Middle Line of vertex, 1. 5 cun in length from Zhengying (GB 17) backward along the Foot-Shaoyang. It belongs to the Gallbladder Meridian of Foot-Shaoyang (See Fig. 6-12). Indications: Contralateral disorders in the shoulders, upper limbs and hands, including paralysis, pain and numbness.

(10) Anterior Temporal Line(MS-10)

Location: From Hanyan(GB 4) to Xuanli(GB 6). It belongs to the Gallbladder Meridian of Foot-Shaoyang (See Fig. 6-12).

Indications: Migraine, peripheral facial paralysis, motor aphasia, and mouth disorders.

(11) Posterior Temporal Line(MS-11)

Location: The line connecting Shuaigu(GB 8) to Qubin(GB 7). It belongs to the Gallbladder Meridian of Foot-Shaoyang (See Fig. 6-12).

Indications: Migraine, dizziness, tinnutis and deafness.

(12) Occipital Upper-Middle Line (MS-12)

Location: The line connecting Qiangjian(DU 18) to Naohu(DU 17). It belongs to the Du Meridian (See Fig. 6-13).

Indications: Lumbar and back pain, eye diseases.

(13) Occipital Upper-lateral Line(MS-13)

Location: 0. 5 cun lateral and parallel to the upper-middle line of the occiput. It belongs to the Bladder Meridian of Foot-Taiyang (See Fig. 6-13).

Indications: Lumbar and back pain, eye diseases. It is often used with the occipital upper-middle line.

(14) Occipital Lower-Lateral Line(MS-14)

Location: The line 2 cun in length from Yuzhen(BL 9) downward to Tianzhu(BL 10). It belongs to the Bladder Meridian of Foot-Taiyang (See Fig. 6-13).

Indications: Equilibrium disorders due to the cerebellum problem, occipital headache.

4. Manipulations and Procedure

(1) Position

The patient should take a sitting or lying posture according to the area selected for puncture. The treating area should be routinely sterilized.

(2) Insertion of the Needle

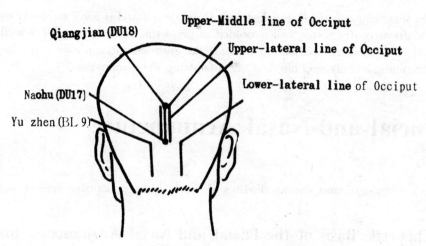

Fig. 6—13 The Puncturing Lines on Occiput Region

Generally, the needle should have a diameter #28-#30 and the length should be from 1. 5 —2. 0 cun. The filiform needle should enter the scalp skin quickly at a 30° angle. The tip of the needle should puncture the deep part of the galea aponeurotica where a decrease in resistance to the needle will be felt. Continue inserting the needle paralle to the skin surface to 0. 5—2. 0 cun in depth.

(3) Operation of the Needle

Use only the twirling method for scalp acupuncture without lifting and thrusting the needle. Avoid changing the depth of needle insertion while twirling. In order to accomplish the twirling easily, the needle is usually held between the palm side of the thumb and the radial side of the index finger and use quick flexion and extension of the metacarpal-phalangeal joint of the index finger to make the needle twirl right and left. The twirling of the needle should be at a rate of 200rpm continuously for two to three minutes. Then, retain the needle for five to ten minutes. Repeat this stimulation procedure two to three times before removing the needle. For hemiplegia, ask the patient to move the affected limbs during the time of needle retention to strengthen the dirigation of the limbs.

(4) Electric Puncture Stimulation

After needle insertion, the practitioner can apply electricd current with a frequency of two to three hundred hertz per minute or higher to replace manual twirling. (For the choice of stimulation wave, refer to the chapter on Electric Acupuncture Therapy.) The stimulation intensity is determined by the patients response.

(5) Treatment Course

Administer once a day or every other day. Ten treatments make a course. Stop treatment for five to seven days before the second course begins.

5. Precautions

(1) During treatment, give the appropriate quantity of stimulation so as to avoid syncope. When the patient is in sitting position, the practitioner should pay special attention to the patient. Observe the patient's face and expression.

(2) Do not use scalp acupuncture for patients who are in acute stage of windstroke with cerebral hemorrhage, coma, fever, or hypertension. However, when the condition and the hypertension of the patient is stable, scalp acupuncture can be done. For hemiparalysis due to cerebral embolism, earliest treatment of scalp puncture combined with body acupuncture may provide very good results. If the patient has a high fever, acute inflammation or heart failure, scalp acupuncture should be used with caution.

(3) The scalp region is richly supplied with blood vessels and is liable to bleed, so when the needle is withdrawn, a dry cotton ball is needed to press the needling hole for a while to avoid bleeding. If bleeding or hematoma occurs after needles are removed, apply soft kneading pressure on the puncture area to help stop bleeding, or dissipating the hematoma.

Ⅲ. Facial and Nasal Acupuncture

This is a method to treat various diseases of the body by puncturing specific points of the face or nose.

1. The Theoretic Basis of the Facial and Nasal Acupuncture and Their Point Distribution Areas

According to the records in *Pivot Miraculous* (灵枢, Ling Su), the face may be divided into different response areas which correspond with diseases of the five Zang and six Fu organs and the limbs. The so-called" By observing the five colors of the face we can determine the type of disease, whether the disease is superficial or deep, acute or chronic; or an area of the body is suffering or not" is an important aspect that the pathogenic changes of the Zang-fu organs and limbs reflect in the superficial. It is also one of the content areas of "learning the condition of the internal organ by observing the changes of the exterior" in the theory of meridian and collateral. The exterior-interior relationship of the Zang-Fu organs with the outside of the body, indicates that certain facial areas may be punctured to treat diseases of the Zang-Fu organs and four limbs.

The nose is in the center of the face. In ancient times it was called "Mingtang". *Pivot Miraculou* (灵枢, Ling Shu) states, "The five colors are reflected in the nose." *Plain Questions* (素问, Su Wen) points out, "The Five Qi enters the nose and is stored in the heart and lung." This means that the nose has a close relationship with the Qi and blood of the whole body and is related with heart and lung functions. According to ancient literature and current clinical practice, practitioners have created facial and nasal acupuncture therapy to treat various diseases of the body. This is a progressive and innovative development from facial inspection to the facial acupuncture.

2. Location and Indications of the Acupoints of Facial acupuncture

Facial acupuncture has seven single points on the nose, forehead and upper lip. The other seventeen points are bilateral such as those around the nose, eyes, mouth, cheek and the zygomatic arch. (See Fig. 6—14) For locations and indications of the facial points, see Tab. 6—2.

3. Location and Indications of the Acupoints of Nosal Acupuncture

Pivot Miraculous (灵枢, Ling Shu) says, "The five Zang are in the center of the nose and six Fu bilateral to the nose⋯." According to this, the nose is divided into three lines with twenty three nasal points. Since the acupoints are named according to the Zang-Fu organs and the indications are characteristic of each Zang-Fu organing, they will not be listed.

Tab. 6-2 Facial Acupoints

Acupoint	Location	Indications
Face	Centre of the forehead	Dizziness, frontal headache
Throat	The mid-point on the line joining the Face and the Lung points	Sore throat
Lung (Yin Tang Ext. 1)	Mid-point between the two inner border of the eyebrows	Cough, stress in the chest
Breast	Mid-point of the line between the Heart point and the inner canthus	Lack of lactation
Heart	The mid-point between the two inner canthus, in the lowest elevation of the bridge of the nose	Palpitation and insomnia
Chest	At the bridge of the nose, at the lower border of the nose bone, where it connects with the nasal cartilage	Chest pain, chest stuffiness
Gallbladder	Directly inferior to the inner canthus, at the same level as the lower border of the nose bridge bone	Nausea, vomiting
Spleen (Suliao Du 25)	Tip of the nose	Poor appetite
Stomach	Both sides of the Spleen point, in the centre of the ala nasi or nasal wing	Stomachache, poor appetite
Uterus, bladder	In the centre of the philtrum	Dysmenorrhea
Small intestine	Lateral to the mid-point between the Gallbladder and the Stomach points	Diarrhea, abdominal pain
Shoulder	Directly inferior to the outer canthus, lateral to the Gall bladder point	Shoulder and arm pain with limitation of movement
Large intestine	Directly inferior to the outer canthus, at the lower border of the zygomatic arch	Constipation, diarrhea
Inner thigh	0. 5 cun lateral to the corner of the mouth where the upper lip joins the lower lip	Pain in the inner aspect of the thigh

Acupoint	Location	Indications
Foot	Directly inferior to the outer canthus at the upper border of the lower jaw	Swollen pain in the foot with limitation of movement
Kidney	At the cross-section of the line horizontally running to the nasal wing and the line running directly inferior to TaiYang (Ext 2), lateral to the Large Intestine point	Scanty, frequent, pain at urination
Umbilicus	0. 3 cun below the Kidney point	Abdominal pain around the umbilicus
Tibia	Anterior to the lower angle of the mandible and on the upper border of the lower jaw	Systremma, swelling of the ankle joint
Arm	At the intersection point of the line directly superior to Xiaguan (St 7), where it meets the lateral line level with the Shoulder point	Swelling and pain of the shoulder and arm
Hand	Directly inferior to the Arm point, at the lower border of the zygomatic arch	Swelling and pain of the hand
Back	1 cun lateral and posterior to the centre of the cheek	Lumbar back pain
Thigh	At the middle and upper one third distance of the line joining the lobe of the ear where it meets with the angle of the lower jaw	Muscle sprain of the thigh
Knee	At the lower and middle one third of the same line as described above for the Thigh point	Swelling pain of the knee joint
Patella	In the depression of the upper border of the lower jaw	Injurg of the knee joint

(1) Basic Nasal Acupoints (See Fig. 6—15).

A. The first line is the central facial line, originating from the centre of the forehead and ending at Shuigou(DU 26), involving nine points or areas. With the exception of the testes and ovaries which are bilateral points, all other points are single points.

B. The second line is the bilateral nostril line, beginning from a point inferior to the inner canthi and descending close to the bridge of the nose, slightly diagonally, to the upper borders of the hostrils . Each bilateral line has five points or areas.

C. The third line is lateral to the second line, originating from the inner canthi and ending at the lower borders of the lateral side of the wings of the nose. Each bilateral line has nine points or areas. For location and indication of nosal acupuncture,(See Tab. 6—3).

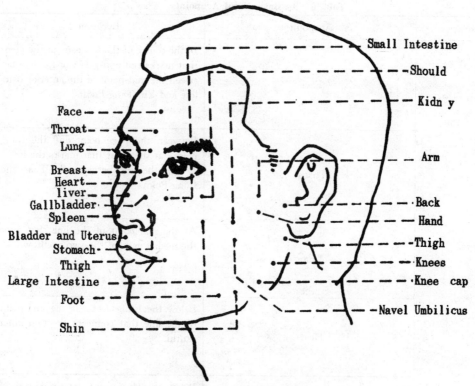

Fig. 6—14   The Acupoints of Facial Acupuncture

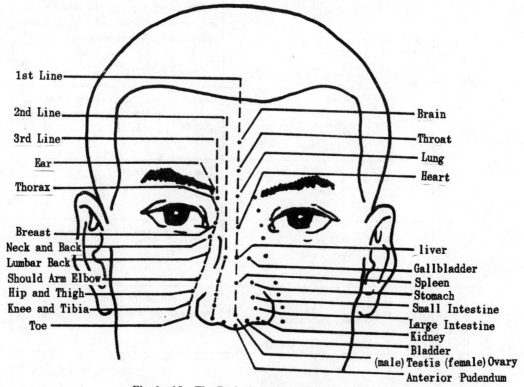

Fig. 6—15   The Basic Acupoints of Nasal Acupuncture

Tab. 6－3 **Basic Nasal Acupoints**

Position	Acupoint	Location
1st line	Face	In the centre of the forhead, at the point that marks the upper 1/3 of the line between the mid-point of the anterior hairline and Yin Tang Point
	Throat	Between the Face point and the Lung point, at the point that marks the lower 1/4 of the line between the Face and Lung Points
	Lung	At the mid-point of the line that joins the medial ends of the two eyebrows
	Heart	Below the Lung area, at the mid-point of the line that connects the two inner canthi
	Liver	Below the Heart area, at the vertex of the nose, at the intersection of the lateral line drawn between the superior border of the zygomatic arch and the longitudinal centre line of the nose
	Spleen	Below the Liver area, on the nasal midline at suliao (Du 25) or the tip of the nose
	Kidney	The tip of the nose
	Ovary-Testes	The area bilateral to the tip of the nose
	Anterior Pudendum	At the end of the inferior border of the septum of the nose

Position	Acupoint	Location
2nd Line	Gall Bladder	Directly inferior to the inner cunthus and lateral to the liver area (point)
	Stomach	Inferior to the Gallbladder and lateral to the Spleen area (point)
	Small Intestine	Inferior to the Stomach area (point) and in the upper 1/3 of the wing of the nose
	Large Intestine	In the centre of the wing of the nose and inferior to the small intestine area
	Bladder	Inferior to the large intestine area, on the border of the wing of the nose
3rd Line	Ear	At the same level as the Lung point and bilaterally at the medial ends of the eyebrows
	Chest	Inferior to the medial ends of the eyebrows, bilaterally on the supraorbital bone
	Breast	The area superior to Jingming (UB 1) point
	Nape and Back area	The area superior to JingMing (UB 1) point
	Spinal and Lumbar area	Lateral to the Gallbladder Point and lateral inferior to the Nape and Back area
	Shoulder, Arm-Hand	The area lateral to the stomach point and lateral inferior to the Lumbar Spinal Point
	Hip and Thigh	Lateral to the superior border of the wing of the nose and inferior to the Shoulder-Arm-Hand Point
	Foot and Toe	Lateral to the inferior border of the wing of the nose and inferior to the Knee Point

(2) New Nasal Acupoints

For the new nasal acupoints. (See Fig. 6—16 and Tab. 6—4)

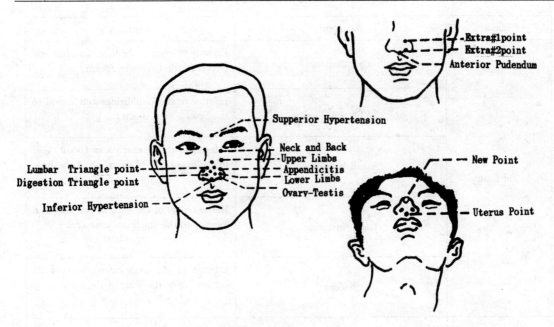

Fig. 6—16 The New Acupoints in the Nose Region

Tab. 6—4 New Nasal Points

Acupoint	Location
Superior Hypertension	The mid-point of the two eyebrows (Yin Tang point)
Lumbar Triangle point	The first point is inferior to the Heart Point The other two points are bilateral to the lower border of the nasal bone
Digestion Triangle point	The first point is inferior to the mid-point of the lumbar Triangle, The other two points are bilateral to the tip of the nose
Inferior Hypertension	Inferior to the tip of the nose
Upper Limbs	Inferior to the nape and back point
Appendix	Lateral and superior to the wing of the nose
Lower Limbs	The same as the Knee and Tibia Point
New point	The point is at the cross-section of the midline of the nose bridge and the lateral line of the superior border of the nostrils
Extra #1 Point	Bilateral points at the inner depression of the wing of the nostrils
Extra #2 point	On a line running from the extra #1 point to the upper border of the nostrils Note: The last three points mentioned can be used for abdominal anesthesia acupuncture
Uterus Point	The point is inferior to the lower border of the nasal septum and superior to Renzhong (Du 26)

4. Manipulations of the Facial and Nasal Acupuncture

Besides treating disease after points are selected based on the diagnosis, facial and nasal acupuncture can be used for acupuncture anesthesia. The concrete manipulation is as follows.

(1) Use a filiform needle #28— #32 in diameter and 0.5—1.5 cun in length. After sterilization, insert the needle to a certain depth according to the location of the acupoints horizontaly, obliquely or perpendicularly. Generally, oblique or horizontal puncture is used for the forehead, nose and mouth areas. Perpendicular insertion is used for the cheek area.

(2) After arrival of Qi (needling sensation), retain the needle twenty to thirty minutes. Then twirl the needle every other five to ten minutes. Embedded needles can also be used when needed. If this kind of acupuncture is used for aneathesia, continuous twirling stimulation is usually required in the forehead, eye and nose areas. Besides, electric acupuncture can be aided in this way.

(3) This is usually done once a day or every other day and ten treatments constitute a single course. The interval between the courses is 5—7 days.

5. Precautions

(1) Strict sterilization procedures must be followed. Avoid bleeding and pain and do not puncture scars.

(2) If using an electric probe to find the sensitive pain areas, first dry the nose with a cotton ball to avoid a false sensitivity reading.

(3) Since the nasal muscle is very thin, the needle to be used should not be too long. In addition, perpendicular insertion is forbidden.

(4) The nasal area is very sensitive, so the insertion of the needle should be mild to relieve pain. Deep insertion or heavy twirling, lifting and thrusting should be avoided.

Ⅳ. Occular Acupuncture

This is a new therapy created by Prof. Peng Jingshan, who followed the theory of "diagnosing diseases by observing the eyes" which was set forth by Huatuo, a physician in the Han Dynasty. The characteristic of this therapy is to select points around the eyes. This therapy has a wide range of indications and especially has a good effect upon the brain and neurological diseases.

1. Occular Distribution Areas

The theory of "diagnosis of diseases by observing the eyes" was expressed by dividing the eyes into eight areas which correspond with the Eight Diagrams(八卦) in Ancient China which were Qian(乾), Kan(坎), Gen(艮), Zhen(震), Xun(巽), Li(离), Kun(坤) and Dui(兑). Prof. Peng Jingshan(彭静山) later renamed these areas respectively from #1 to #8. The left eye is numbered in a clockwise direction and the right eye in an anti-clockwise direction.

For acupoint distribution, (See Fig. 6—17).

Area 1: Lung and Large Intestine

Area 2: Kidney and Bladder

Area 3: Upper Jiao

Area 4: Liver and Gallbladder

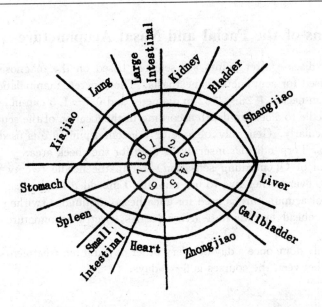

**Fig. 6—17   The Distribution of Acupoint of Areas of
Occular Acupuncture**

Area 5: Middle Jiao
Area 6: Heart and Small Intestine
Area 7: Spleen and Stomach
Area 8: Lower Jiao

This system uses eight areas involving thirteen points to summarize the organs of the whole body. All the points are located 0.2 cun interiorly from the border of the orbital foramen, which are termed as "orbital area and acupoints of the eyes".

2. Manipulation and Procedure

Use sterile filiform needles #30 — #32 in diameter and 0.5 cun in length. Press the orbit closely and insert the needle slowly. The puncture can be done perpendicularly, subcutaneosly (i. e. horizontally) or obliquely to the periosteum. Puncture in the hypodermal skin 0.2 to 0.3 cun in depth, and allow the needle to remain in the designated area without any manipulation. If there is no arrival of Qi(needling sensation), withdraw the needle and repeat the puncture. The time for retaining the needle is five to thirty minutes. It is important to follow strict sterilization procedures before and after the needling to prevent infection. When withdrawing the needle, use a dry cotton ball to apply pressure to the hole to avoid bleeding or hematoma due to accidental injury of the veins and arteries. The practitioner should take care to protect the eyeball and eyelid. When puncturing the inner canthus, deep puncture is forbidden so as to avoid injuring the artery.

3. Acupoints Selection

(1) Selecting points according to different occular areas
Observe the occular areas based on the disease and note any changes of shape and color in the blood vessels in the bulbar conjunctiva. If there is any change, the points are selected in the corresponding area.

(2) Selecting points according to the eyes
If there occurs any obvious changes of the blood vessels in the occular area, no matter what disease it is, puncture the corresponding acupoints in this area.

(3) Selecting points according to the location of the disease.

Based on the different location of the disease in the upper, middle and lower Jiao, select the corresponding points of the respective jiao.

(4) Indications

Generally, all the diseases which can be treated with body acupuncture and moxibustion can be treated by testing this occular acupuncture therapy. All the diseases of the whole body may be treated by this therapy. It has an especially good effect on diseases of the nervous system, pain diseases and brain diseases. When this therapy is used, strict sterilization procedures must be followed and care must be taken to avoid bleeding and he, atomas.

V. **Wrist and Ankle Acupuncture**

This therapy was summarized and created by the Neurology Department of the First Teaching Hospital attached to the Second Military Medical University in Xi'an, China. Its characteristic is that there are twenty four needle-entering points in all of the four limbs which are all located at the wrist and ankle areas. The puncturing technique involves inserting the needle to the depth of the hypodermis. No sensation is required to get good results. In fact, less the sensation, the better the effect.

(1) Manipulation

The patient can take any position convenient for treatment. If puncturing the ankles, it is preferable for the patient to lie down. Use sterile filiform needles #30 in diameter and 1.5 cun in length. Insert the needle subcutaneously and obliquely. No manipulation and needling sensation is required.

The characteristic of this therapy is to divide the head, trunk and the four limbs into different areas according to the anatomical standard of the bones. (See Fig. 6—18, 6—19, 6—20).

(2) Points for Needle Insertion

There are six points located at the circle about two finger-breradths proximal to the transverse crease of the wrist, three on the palmar aspect and three on the dorsal aspect of the wrist. They are, in order, termed upper 1—6 from the ulnar side to the radial side of the palmar surface and then from the radial side to the ulnar side of the dorsal surface. (See Fig. 6—21).

Upper #1 Point: In the depression of the palmar aspect of the medial border of the ulnar.

Upper #2 Point: The same as Neiguan (PC 6), but 2 transverse fingers above the wrist crease instead of 2 cun.

Upper #3 Point: Lateral aspect of the radial artery, along the lung meridian, 2 transverse fingers above the wrist fold.

Upper #4 Point: With the thumb facing upwards on the lateral aspect of the radial bone on the dorsal aspect, 2 transverse fingers above the wrist fold.

Upper #5 Point: Same as Waiguan (SJ 5), but 2 transverse fingers above the wrist crease instead of 2 cun. Between the radius and the ulna the dorsel aspect with the palm facing downwards.

Upper #6 Point: With the palm facing downwards, on the dorsal aspect medial to the ulnar bone, along the small intestine Meridian, 2 transverse fingers above the wrist fold.

There are a total of six points located on the wrist. The posture of the hand to puncture will affect the location, so it is very important the location be in the correct position.

The acupoints in the ankle area are located at the circle about three finger-breadths proximal to the highest points of internal and external condyles, with three points on the lateral side and three on the medial side of the leg. They are termed lower 1-6 in order circling the ankle from the internal side to the external side of the Achilles tendon. There are a total of six points on the an-

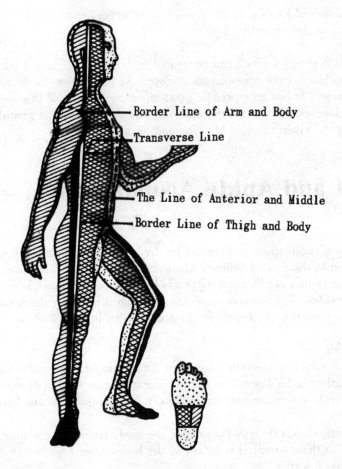

Border Line of Arm and Body

Transverse Line

The Line of Anterior and Middle

Border Line of Thigh and Body

Fig. 6—18   The Areas of Body Laterior of the Wrist and Ankle Acupuncture Therapy

kle. To puncture the ankle, choose a lying posture to relax the muscles. (See Fig. 6—22).

Lower #1 Point: On the interior border of the Achilles tendon, 3 transverse fingers above the medial malleolus.

Lower #2 Point: On the posterior border of the tibia, 3 transverse fingers above the medial malleolus.

Lower #3 Point: On the posterior border of the tibia and 1cm posterior to the anterior creast of the tibia, 3 transverse fingers above the medial malleolus.

Lower #4 Point: Mid-point between the anterior border of the fibula and lateral border of the anterior crast of the tibia, 3 transverse fingers above the lateral malleolus.

Lower #5 Point: At the center of the lateral side, 3 transverse fingers above the lateral malleolus near the posterior border of the fibia

Lower #6 Point: On the anterior border of the Achilles tendon on the lateral aspect of the leg, 3 transverse fingers above the lateral malleolus.

(3) Principle of Needle Insertion

Puncture the acupoints of the wrist or ankle based on the different affected areas. i. e. if the diseasesd area is on the right side of the body, the points on the right wrist and ankle are punctured; and if the diseased area is on the left side, the points on the left wrist and ankle are punctured. Likewise, if the diseased area is above the diaphragm, the wrist area is punctured. If the diseased area is below the diaphragm, the ankle area is punctured. If the disease is in the frontal aspect of the body, the points of the palmar aspect of the wrist or the medial aspect of the ankle

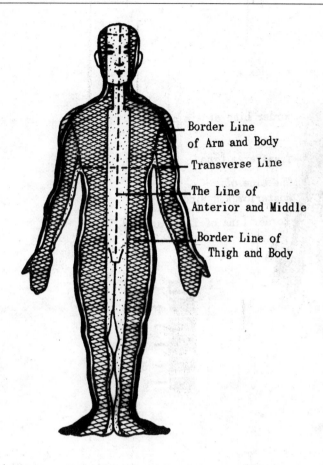

**Border Line
of Arm and Body**

Transverse Line

**The Line of
Anterior and Middle**

**Border Line of
Thigh and Body**

**Fig. 6—19 The Areas of Body Anteriorof the Wrist and Ankle
Acupuncture Therapy**

are punctured. And if the disease is in the dorsal aspect of the body, the points of the dorsal side of the wrist or the lateral side of the ankle are punctured. When selecting the inserting point, first observe the disease focus, and then, according to the focus, determine which area will receive the needle. The choice of the acupoints should be based on the main symptoms of the disease. Sometimes only one point is used and sometimes several points are needed.

(4) Clinical Applications

This therapy has a good effect on various pain diseases.

VI. Hand and Foot Acupuncture

This is a method to treat diseases by using specific points on the hand and foot.

(1) The Relationship between Foot, Hand and the Zang-Fu organs and Meridian-Collateral System

In *Yellow Emperor's Internal Classic*(黄帝内经, Huang Di Nei Jing,) it is recorded that the four limbs have a general relationship through the meridians and collaterals with both Zang-Fu organs and whole body. *Pivot Miraculous*(灵枢, Ling Shu)says, "The hand and foot collaterals are like big collaterals for qi with the Yang Meridians collecting there. The qi of the twelve sub-

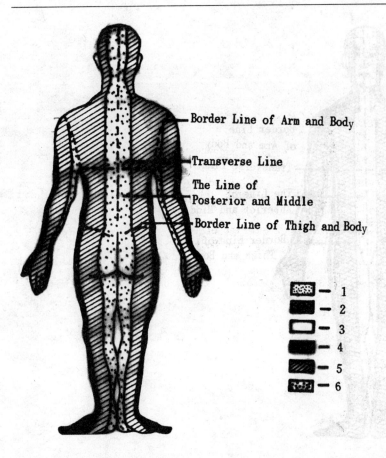

Border Line of Arm and Body

Transverse Line

The Line of
Posterior and Middle

Border Line of Thigh and Body

1
2
3
4
5
6

Fig. 6—20   The Areas of Body Posterior of the Wrist and Ankle Acupuncture Therapy

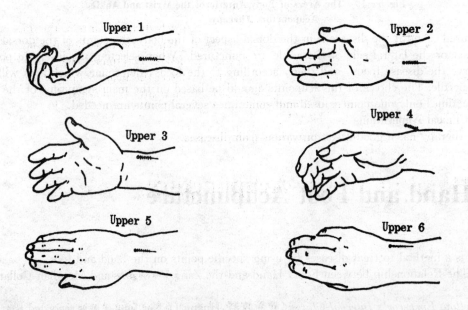

Upper 1

Upper 2

Upper 3

Upper 4

Upper 5

Upper 6

Fig. 6—21   The Locations for Insertion on the Wrist

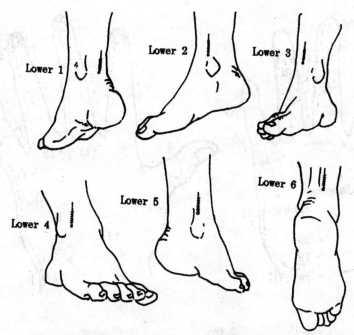

Fig. 6—22   **The Locations for Insertion on the Ankle**

cutaneous regions gathers in the hand and feet, which indicates that the Yin and Yang Meridians of foot and hand are the gathering areas of the qi and blood. Puncturing the different points of the hand and foot can treat diseases of the whole body.

(2) Location and Indications of the Hand Points

The palm division and the distribution of the Zang-Fu Organ areas on the palms are as follows: (See Fig. 6—23, 6—24, See Tab. 6—5).

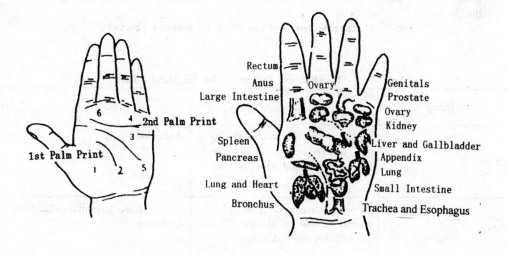

Fig. 6—23   **The Distributed Areas of the Palm**

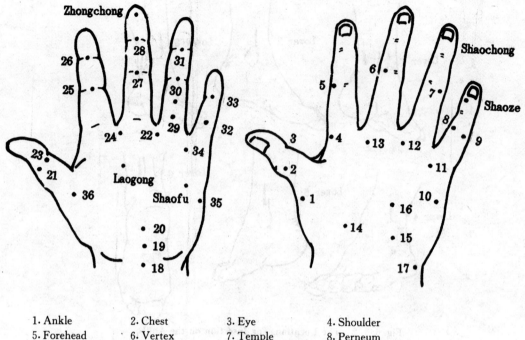

1. Ankle   2. Chest   3. Eye   4. Shoulder
5. Forehead   6. Vertex   7. Temple   8. Perneum
9. Occiput   10. Spine   11. Sciatic Nerve
12. Throat   13. Neck   14. 1st Lumbus and Thigh
15. 2nd Lumbus and Thigh   16. Coccyx   17. Antipruritic Point
18. Arresting Convulsion   19. Foot   20. Stomach and Intestine
21. Chest Pain   22. Toothache   23. Spleen
24. Asthma   25. Large Intestine   26. Small Intestine
27. Sanjiao   28. Heart   29. Gallbladder   30. Liver
31. Lung   32. Mingmen   33. Kidney   34. New Point of Asthma
35. Bladder   36. Larynx

Fig. 6—24   The Acupoints of the Hand Acupuncture Therapy

Tab. 6—5   Location and Indications for the Hand Points

Acupoint	Location	Indications
Ankle	At the metacarpophalangeal joint of the thumb on the radial aspect where the red and white skin meet	Ankle joint pain
Chest	At the phalangeal joint of the thumb on the radial aspect where the red and white skin meet	Chest pain, vomit, diarrhea, dysentery.
Edema	At the ulnar aspect of the thumb nail 0.1 cun from the comen of the nail bed	Eye diseases: conjunctivitis lacrimation, sty

Acupoint	Location	Indications
Superior HeGu	On the dorsal aspect of the hand, at the junction of the thumb and index finger metacarpal bones	Neurosis, headache due to nerves, trigeminal neuralgia, schizophrenia, hypertention, hemiparalysis, sequela of infantile paralysis
Shoulder	At the radial aspect of the index finger at the metacarpalphalangeal joint where the red and white skin meet	Shoulder pain
Forehead (Appendicitis)	At the proximal phalangeal joint on the radial aspect of the index finger where the red and white skin meet	Frontal headache, gastric spasm, acute gastroenteritis, early stage of acute appendicitis
Ear	On the dorsal aspect of the hand, in the centre of the metacarpalphalangeal joint of the index finger	Otogenic dizzyness, deafness, tinnitus
Breast	On the dorsal aspect of the hand, at the radial side of the phalangeal joint of the middle finger where the red and white skin meets	Headache due to nerves, headache at the vertex, dysmenorrhea
Lateral Head	On the ulnar aspect of the proximal phalangeal joint of the ring finger where the red and white skin meets	Migraine, intercostal neuralgia, hypochondrac pain, ear pain
HuiYin	On the ulnar aspect of the proximal phalangeal joint of the little finger where the red and white skin meets	Pain in the perineum, dysmenorrhea, profuse leukorrhea
Posterior Head (Tonsil)	On the ulnar aspect of the distal phalangeal joint of the little finger where the red and white skin meets	Posterior headache, tonsilitis, spinal column pain, popliteal fossa pain
Spinal Column (Coccyx Pain Point)	On the ulnar aspect of the metacarpalphalangeal joint of the little finger where the red and white skin meets	Acute lumbar sprain, prolapse of lumbar vertebral disc, coccyx pain
Sciatic Nerve	On the dorsum of the hand between the fourth and fifth metacarpalphalangeal joints the medial side	Hip joint pain, buttock pain
Nose	On the dorsum of the hand, in the centre of the metacarpalphalangeal joint of the ring finger	Nose disease

Acupoint	Location	Indications
Throat	On the dorsum of the hand, between the third and the fourth metacarpalphalangeal joint, but closer to the third metaearpalphalangeal joint	Acute tonsilitis, sorethroat, toothache, trigeminal neuralgia
Neck and Nape	On the dorsum of the hand, between the second and third metacarpalphalangeal joint but closer to the third	Stiff neck, cervical muscle sprain
Pericardium	On the dorsum of the hand, on the metacarpalphalangeal joint of the index finger, half way between the midpoint of the joint and it's extreme ulnar aspect	Coma, delirium due to febrile disease
#1 Lumbar Leg	On the dorsum of the hand, 1.5 cun anterior to the carpal cross striation, on the radial aspect of the second extensor tendon	Lumbar leg pain, lumbar sprain, treat the hand of the affected side
#2 Lumbar Leg	On the dorsum of the hand, in the depression anterior to the meeting of the metacarpal bones of the little finger and the ring finger	Lumbar leg pain, lumbar sprain, inflammation of the urethra, nephritis, pain due to Kidney stones
Stop Bleeding	On the dorsum of the hand, where the metacarpal bone of the ring finger meets the transverse wrist crease	Any type of hemorrage
Hyperthyroidism	On the dorsum of the hand, where the metacarpal bone of the little finger meets the transverse wrist crease in the depression anterior to the ulnar bone	Hyperthyroidism
Sacrum	On the lateral aspect of the metacarpal bone of the little finger, where it meets with the transverse wrist crease	Soreness and pain of the sacrum
Antipuritic	1 cun anterior to the transverse wrist crease on the ulnar aspect of the wrist, where the red and white skin meets	Puritis, neural dermatitis, urticaria

Acupoint	Location	Indications
Hip	On the dorsum of the hand towards the ulnar aspect of the mid-point of the metacarpal bone of the little finger	Hip area pain
Mouth	On the dorsum of the hand, in the centre of the metacarpalphalangral joint of the little finger	Stomatologic diseases
Increase Blood Pressure	On the dorsum of the hand, in the middle of the transverse wrist crease	Hypotension
Decrease Blood Pressure	On the dorsum of the hand, 0.5 cun posterior to the ulnar aspect of the metacarpalphalangeal joint of the index finger	Hypertension
Hiccup	On the dorsum of the hand, in the mid-point of the distal phalangeal joint of the middle finger	Hiccup
Reduce Fever	On the dorsum of the hand, on the radial aspect of the web between the middle finger and the ring finger	Fever, diarrhea, occular disease
Diarrhea Point	On the dorsum of the hand, 1 cun superior to the mid-point between the third and fourth metacarpalphalangeal joint	Diarrhea
Calm the Spirit	On the palm of the hand, where the big thenar eminence and the small thenar eminence meets	High fever, convulsion
Heel	At the mid-point on the line, between the stomach-Intestine point and Daling Point (PC. 7)	Heel pain
Stomach-Intestine	On the palm of the hand, at the mid-point between Laogong (PC. 8) and Daling (PC. 7)	Chronic gastritis, alimentary ulcer, indigestion, biliary ascariasis
Chest Pain	On the palmar aspect of the thumb on the radiao one third of the phalangeal crease	Chest depression, chest pain, intercostal neuralgia

Acupoint	Location	Indications
Toothache	On the palmar aspect of the hand, between the third and fourth metacarpalphalangeal joint	Toothache, throat disease
Spleen	On the palmar aspect of the thumb, at the mid-point of the phalangeal crease	Indigestion, abdominal pain, diarrhea
Asthma	On the palmar aspect of the hand, to the ulnar side of the mid-point of the metacarpalphalangeal joint of the index finger	Bronchitis, asthma, neural headache, stiff neck
Large Intestine	On the palmar aspect of the hand, at the mid-point of the proximal phalangeal crease of the index finger	Diarrhea, constipation
Small Intestine	On the palmar aspect of the hand, at the mid-point of the distal phalangeal crease of the index finger	Small intestine disease
SanJiao	On the palmar aspect of the hand, at the mid-point of the proximal phalangeal crease of the middle finger	Chest disease, abdominal and pelvic cavity disease
Heart (Infantile Digestion)	On the palmar aspect of the hand, at the mid-point of the distal phalangeal crease of the middle finger	palpitation, cardiac pain, neurasthenia, infantile indigestion, asthma, urticaria, vitiligo(use moxa)
Liver	On the palmar aspect of the hand, at the mid-point of the proximal phalangeal crease of the ring finger	Liver and gallbladder diseases, hyperchondiac pain, fullness distention in the epigastrium
Lung	On the palmar aspect of the hand, at the mid-point of the distal phalangeal crease of the ring finger	Cough, depression of the chest
Ming Men	On the palmar aspect of the hand, at the mid-point of the phoximal phalangeal crease of the little finger	Lumbago, nocturnal emission, impotence
Kidney	On the palmar aspect of the hand, at the distal phalangeal crease of the little finger	Nocturia

Acupoint	Location	Indications
New Asthma Point	On the palmar aspect of the hand, in the anterior depression between the fourth and fifth metacarpal-phalangeal joints or 0.3 cun posterior to the web where the red and white skin meets, between the metacarpal bones	Asthma
Insomnia	On the dorsum of the hand, at the mid-point of the line joining Hegu (LI. 4)and SanJian (LI. 3)	Insomnia
Pelvic cavity	On the palmar aspect of the hand, at the mid-point of the middle phalangeal bone of the middle finger	Abdominal and pelvic cavity disease, influenza
Uterus point	On the palmar aspect of the hand, at the mid-point of a line drawn from the point where the tip of the little finger rests against the ring finger and running between the fourth and fifth metacarpal bones to the transverse wrist crease	Reproductive system disease
Malaria	On the ulnar aspect of the large thenar eminence where the first metacarpal bone meets at the transverse wrist crease	Malaria
YuJi (Tonsil #2)	On the palmar aspect of the hand, at the mid-point of the ulnar aspect of the first metacarpal bone	Tonsilitis, laryngitis

A. For the location and indication of the basic points of the sole of the foot, see Fig. 6—25 and Tab. 6—6.

B. For the basic points of the dorsum of the foot, see Tab. 6—7.

C. For the basic points of the medial aspects of the foot, see Tab. 6—8.

D. For the new points of the foot, see Fig. 6—26 and Tab. 6—9.

(3) Location and Indications of the Foot Points

For convenience, the proportional measurements of the foot are made as follows:

First, on the sole aspect of the foot, a line drawn from the mid-point of the posterior border of the heel to the mid-point between the second and third toes which is 10 cun in length.

Second, the distance between the two lines that run perpendicularly from the mid-parts of the malleolus, both medial and lateral, to the sole of the foot, which is 3 cun across the sole of the foot.

Third, the widest distance of the heel across the sole of the foot which is 3 cun in length.

Fourth, the distance between each parallel line from each toe to the heel which is 1 cun in length.

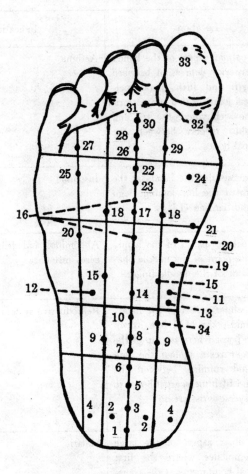

1. Head   2. Eye   3. Nose   4. Ear
5. Mouth   6. Throat   7. Zaisheng   8. Heart
9. Lung   10. Anmian   11. Liver   12. Spleen
13. Gallbladder   14. Stomach   15. Small Intestine

16. Anterior and Posterior-Yinzhu
17. Yongquan (KI. 1) 18. Kidney   19. No. 1 Root of Cancer
20. Large Intestine   21. Gongsun (SP4)   22. Genitals
23. Bladder   24. No. 2 Root of Cancer   25. Nei Linqi
26. Li Xiangu   27. Nei Xiaxi   28. Anus
29. Nei Taichong   30. Li Neiting
31. Duyin   32. Dazhili Hengwen   33. Qiduan
34. No. 3 Root of Cancer

Fig. 6－25   Basic Acupoints of the Sole Aspect of the Foot

Tab. 6—6 **Location and Indications of the Basic Points of the Sole Aspect of the Foot**

Point	Location	Indications
Head	I cun anterior to the midpoint of the dorso-ventral boundary of the foot which is close to the heel, on the middle line	Headache
Nose	I cun anterior to the pt. Head, directly towards the heel and pt. Head, on the middle line	Acute and chronic rhinitis
Ear	1. 2 cun lateral to pt. Nose	Tinnutis, deafness
Mouth	I cun anterior to pt. Nose, on the middle line	Toothache, pharyngitis, tonsillitis
Zaisheng	0. 6 cun anterior to Pt. Larynx, on the middle line	Relieve pain and improve symptoms for the tumor of the intracranial part and spinal cord. The tip of needle is towards both sides of the heel
Larynx	0. 6 cun anterior to pt. Mouth, on the middle line	Fever, pharyngitis, tonsillitis, common cold
Heart	0. 5 cun anterior to pt. Zaisheng, on the middle line	Hypertension, cardiac failure, laryngitis, tongue inflammation, insomnia, dream disturbed sleep
Lung	There are two points, I cun lateral and 0. 1 cun slightly posterior to pt. Heart	Cough, asthma, chest pain
Anmian	0. 6 cun anterior to pt. Heart, on the middle line	Neurosis, schizophrenia, hysteria
Stomach	0. 8 cun anterior to pt. Anmian, on the middle line	Gastric pain, vomiting, indigestion
Liver	1. 2 cun medial to pt. Stomach	Chronic hepatites, cholecystitis, eye problem; intercostal neuralgia
Spleen	1. 2 cun lateral to pt. Stomach	Indigestion, retention of urine, hematopathy
Gallbladder	0. 3 cun posterior to Pt. Liver, directly below Pt. Liver	Cholecystits, hypochondrium
Small intestine	2 points, each I cun lateral and 0. 3 cun anterior to Pt. Stomach, directly superior to Pt. Lung	Borborygmus, abdominal pain

Point	Location	Indications
Anterior and posterior Yinzhu	Pt. Anterior Yinzhu is 0. 4 cun anterior to Yongquan (K1), Pt. posterior Yinzhu is 0. 6 cun posterior to Yongquan, both of them are on the middle line	Hypertention, schizophrenia, epilepsy, high fever, coma
Yongquan (K1)	approximately at the junction of the anterior and middle third of the sole	Hypertention, vertex pain, infantile convulsion, shock, epilepsy
Kidney	2 points, each I cun lateral to Pt. Yongquan	Hypertention, schizophrenia, acute lumbago, retention of urine
No. 1 Aigen	I cun anterior and superior to Pt. liver	Relieve pain and improve symptoms for a tumor of the stomach, cardiac orifice and lower segment of esophagus. When stimulating, the tip of the needle is better towards Yongquan (K1), Rangu (K2) Gongsun (Sp 4) and Anmian
Large intestine	Pt. Medial large intestine is located at 1. 2 cun medial and 0. 2 cun posterior to Pt. Posterior Yinzhu. Pt. lateral large intestine at 2 cun lateral, 0. 2 cun posterior to Pt. Posterior Yinzhu	Abdominal pain, diarrhea, functional disorder of large intestine
Gongsun (Sp. 4)	In the depression of the boundary between the white and red colored skin, anterior to the base of the 1st metatarsal bone	Stomachache, vomiting, abdominal distention, indigestion
Bladder	I cun anterior to Yongquan (K1), on the middle line	Retention of urine, neuresis, urinary incontinence
Genitals	0. 3 cun anterior to Pt. Bladder	Irregular menstruation, profuse leukorrhea, testitis, impotence, retention of ruine
No. 2 Aigen	2 cun medial and 0. 1 cun anterior to Pt. Bladder	Relieve pain and improve symptoms for the cancer of lymphoid transfer and the tumor of visceral organs below the umbilicus. The tip of needle is towards Gongsun (Sp. 4), Yongquan (K1) and Pt. No. 1 Aigen when stimulating
Nei linqi	the corresponding point to the palm aspect of Zu Linqi (GB. 41), on the middle line	Migrain, hypochondrium pain, eye problem, tinnutis, deafness, fever.

Point	Location	Indications
Li Xiangu	the Corresponding point to the palm aspect of Xiangu (St. 43), on the middle line	Acute stomachache, indigestion, schizophrenia
Anus	0.6 cun anterior to Pt. Li xiangu	Diarrhea, constipation
Nei Taichong	The corresponding point to the palm aspect of Taichong (Liv. 3)	Testitis, hernial pain, dysfunctional uterine bleeding, irregular menstruation, profuse leukorrhea, dysmenorrhea, hypochondric pain, schizophrenia, hepatitis, hypertention, eye problem
Li Neiting	The corresponding point to the palm aspect of Neiting (St. 44), on the middle line	Infantile convulsion
Du Yin	The midpoint of the cross striation below the 2nd toe	Hernia, irregular menstruation, retention of placenta
Dai zhi Li Heng Wen	The midpoint of the cross striation below the big toe	Testitis, hernial pain
No. 3 Aigen	0.6 cun anterior to the medial aspect of Pt. Lung	Relieve pain and improve symptoms for the tumor of the upper and middle segment of esophagus, lung, neck, nose and throat
Qiduan	The tip of the toe	Beriberi, numbness of toes, obstructive phlebitis

Tab. 6－7　Location and Indications of the Basic Point of the Dorsum Aspect of the Foot

Point	Location	Indications
Headache Point	Medial side of the boundary of white and red colored skin between the 2nd and the 3rd toes on the dorsum aspect of the foot	Headache
Tonsil 1	Medial side of the tendon of long extensor muscle of toe, at the metatarsophalangeal joint of the foot	Tonsillitis, epidemic mumps, eczema, urticaria
Tonsil 2	The midpoint of the line connecting Taichong (Liv. 3) and Xingjian (Liv. 2)	Acute tonsillitis, acute mumps
Lumbago point	The depression at the lateral and anterior aspect of the little head of the 1st metatarsal bone	Acute lumbar sprain, lumbago

Point	Location	Indications
Ischium 2	The midpoint of the line connecting Zulinqi (GB. 41) and Diwuhui (GB. 42), on the dorsum aspect of the foot	Sciatica
Stiff neck	2 cun posterior to the web between the 3rd and the 4th of the toes, on the dorsum aspect of the foot	Stiff neck
Gastric-intestine point	3 cun posterior to the web between the 2nd and the 3rd of the toes, on the dorsum aspect of the foot	Acute and chronic gastroenteritis, gastroduodenal ulcer
Cardiac pain point	2.5 cun inferior to Jiexi (St. 41)	Cardiac pain, palpitation, cardiac asthma, common cold
Lumbus and leg Point	Two points 0.5 cun inferior to Jiexi (St. 41), at the depressions on the left and right aspect	Pain in lumbar region and leg, spasm and pain in lower limbs

Tab. 6—8 **Location and Indications of the Basic Points of the Medial Aspect of the Foot**

Point	Location	Indications
Dizziness point	The depression superior to the high prominnece of the navicular bone, on the medial aspect of the foot	Dizziness, headache, hypertention, epidemic mumps, acute tonsillitis
Dysmenorrhea 1	2 cun directly inferior to the tip of the medial malleolus	Dysfunctional uterine bleeding, irregular menstruation, dysmenorrhea
Dysmenorrhea 2	The depression inferior to the tuberosity of the navicular bone, the medial aspect of the foot	Dysmenorrhea, dysfunctional uterine bleeding, annexitis
Epilepsy point	The midpoint of the line connecting Taibai (Sp. 3) and Gongsun (Sp. 4)	Epilepsy, hysteria, nerosism
Arm	I cun directly superior to Kunlun (BL. 60)	Sciatica, headache, abdominal pain

Tab. 6—9 **New Point of the Foot**

Point	Location	Indications
No. 1	I cun directly superior to the the mid-point of the posterior border of the sole aspect of the foot	Common cold, headache, maxillary si-nusitis, rhinitis
No. 2	3 cun directly superior and I cun medial to the midpoint of the posterior border of the sole aspect of the foot	Trigeminal neuralgia
No. 3	3 cun directly superior to the midpoint of the posterior border of the sole aspect of the foot (the midpoint of the line connecting the lateral malleolus and medial one of the sole aspect of the foot)	Neurosism, hysteria, insonmia, hypotension, coma
No. 4	3 cun directly superior and I cun lateral to the midpoint of the posterior border of the sole aspect of the foot	Intercostal neuralgia, chest distress, chest pain
No. 5	4 cun directly superior and 1. 5 cun lateral to the midpoint of the posterior border of the sole aspect of the foot	Sciatica, appendicitis, chest pain
No. 6	5 cun directly superior and 1 cun lateral to the midpoint of the posterior border of the sole aspect of the foot	Dysentery, diarrhea, duodenal ulcer
No. 7	5 cun directly superior to the midpoint of the posterior border of the sole aspect of the foot	Asthma, maldevelopment of brain
No. 8	I cun lateral to Pt. No. 7	Neurosism, epilepsy, neurosis
No. 9	4 cun posterior to the midpoint of the big toe and the 2nd toe	Dysentery, diarrhea, uteritis
No. 10	I cun medial and lateral to Yongquan (K1)	Chronic gastroenteritis, gastric spasm
No. 11	2 cun medial and lateral to Yongquan (K1)	Shoulder pain, urticaria
No. 12	1 cun directly superior to the midpoint of the anterior border of the sole of the foot	Toothache
No. 13	1 cun posterior to the midpoint of the cross striation of the big toe of the sole aspect of the foot	Toothache

Point	Location	Indications
No. 14	The midpoint of the cross striation of the little toe	Neuresis, frequently urine
No. 15	The two depressions 0. 5 cun lateral to the midpoint of the cross striation of the malleolus joint	Loin and leg pain, systremma
No. 16	The depression superior to the tubercle of the navicular bone of the lateral aspect of the foot	Hypertention, epidemic mumps, acute tonsillitis
No. 17	2. 5 cun inferior to the midpoint of the cross striation of the malleolus joint	Angina pectoris, asthma, common cold
No. 18	The depression anterior-medial to the head of the lst metatarsal bone on the dorsum aspect of the foot	Chest pain, chest stress, acute lumbar sprain
No. 19	3 cun posterior to the middle of the 2nd and 3rd toes on the dorsum aspect of the foot	Headache, tympanitis, acute and chronic gastroenteritis, gastroduodenal ulcer
No. 20	2 cun posterior to the middle of the 3rd and 4th toes on the dorsum aspect of the foot	Stiff neck
No. 21	0. 5 cun posterior to the middle of the 4th and 5th toes on the dorsum of the foot	Sciatica, epidemic mumps, tonsillitis
No. 22	1 cun posterior to the middle of the 1st and 2nd toes on the dorsum of the foot	Acute tonsillitis, epidemic mumps, hypertention
No. 23	At the metatarsophalangeal joint, medial to the tendon of long extensor muscle of great toe	Acute tonsillitis, epidemic mumps, hypertension, prurigo nodularis, eczema, urticaria
No. 24	The bundary of white and red colored skin, medial to the 2nd joint of the 2nd toe	Headache, tympanitis
No. 25	The bundary of white and red colored skin, medial to the 2nd joint of the 3rd toe	Headache

Point	Location	Indications
No. 26	The bundary of white and red colored skin, medial to the 2nd joint of the 4th toe	Headache, hypotention
No. 27	The midpoint of the line connecting Taibai (Sp. 3) and Gongsun (Sp. 4)	Epilepsy, hysteria, abdominal pain
No. 28	The depression posterior to the high prominnence of the navicular bone on the medial aspect of the foot	Dysmenorrhea, dysfunction uterine bleeding, trachitis, asthma
No. 29	2 cun directly inferior to the middle of the medial malleolus	Dysfunction uterine bleeding, trachitis, atsthma
No. 30	1. 5 cun posterior superior to the lateral malleolus	Sciatica, lumbago, headache

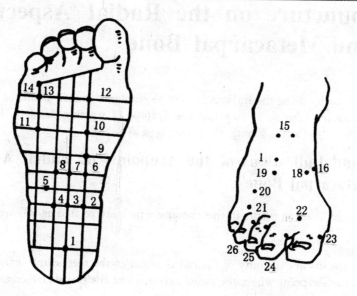

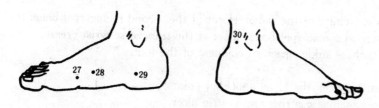

Fig. 6 – 26 New Points of the Foot

(4) Manipulations of the Hand and Foot Acupuncture

A. Use sterile filiform needle #28 to #32 in diameter and 1.0 to 2.0 cun in length. After sterilization, puncture obliquely or perpendicularly 0.3 to 0.5 cun in depth. Use moderate or strong stimulation. Retain the needle three to five minutes.

B. When puncturing the Lumbar-Leg points on the hand, insert the needle obliquely at 15 to 30 angle towards the palm between the extensor tendon and metacarpal bone to a depth of 0.5 to 0.8 cun.

C. To treat the injury of lumbar region or soft tissues, ask the patient to move about or massage the affected area while the needle is being twirled and stimulated.

D. After the pain is relieved, when treating pain diseases, continue stimulation by further twirling the needle for one to three minutes. Sometimes, prolongation of retaining needles or embedded needle therapy is necessary. For patients who need continuous stimulations, electric acupuncture can be used.

(5) Precautions

When using hand and foot acupuncture, the practitioner should explain to the patient that this kind of therapy prorides strong stimula tion. The patient should be mentally prepared to avoid the possible occurrence of acupuncture syncope. When puncturing obliquely close to the bone, take care not to damage the periosteum. Careful sterilization procedures must be followed, specially in the foot, as infection can easily occur in this area.

VII. Acupuncture on the Radial Aspect of the Second Metacarpal Bone

This is a therapy by using the filiform needles to stimulate specific points of the radial aspect of the second metacarpal bone so as to attain the purpose of treating diseases. This method was first created in 1980's by Doctor Zhang Yingqing(张颖清).

1. Location and Indications of the Acupoints of Radial Aspect of the Second Metacarpal Bone

There are a total of seven points in this therapy which are related as follows: (See Fig. 6—27).

(1) Head Point

Location: At the distal extremity of the radial aspect of the second metacarpal bone. When a loose fist is made, it is the point where the radial extremity of the transverse crease of the palm intersects with the second metacarpal bone.

Indications: Face and head diseases, as well as neurotic disorders and other mental diseases.

(2) Foot Point

Location: At the proximal extremity of the radial aspect of the second metacarpal bone. It is the point where the first and second metacarpal bones meet at the transverse wrist crease.

Indications: Foot diseases such as ankle sprain or coldness of the foot.

(3) Stomach Point

Location: At the mid-point between the Head and Foot points.

Indications: Gastric diseases such as gastritis and gastric ulcer.

(4) Lung Point

Location: At the mid-point between the Head and the Stomach points.

Indications: Lung and heart diseases.

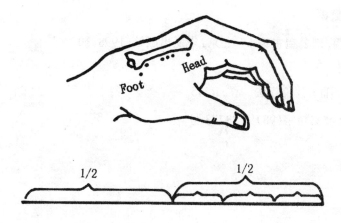

Fig. 6—27 The Acupoints of Acupuncture of the Radial Aspect of the Second Metacarpal Bone

(5) Liver Point

Location: At the mid-point between the Lung and Stomach points.

Indications: Liver and gallbladder diseases.

(6) Umbilicus Point

Location: On the line connecting the Stomach and Foot points, at 1/3 the distance close to the Stomach point.

Indications: Diseases of the trunk and Zang-Fu organs manifested in the periumbilical area such as diarrhea and abdominal pain.

(7) Lumbar Point

Location: On the line connecting the Stomach Point and the Foot Point, at 1/3 the distance from the Foot point.

Indications: Urinary Bladder and Kidney disorders, uterine bleeding and dismenorshea, wrist problems.

2. Manipulations of the Acupuncture of the Radial Aspect of the Second Metacarpal Bone

After locating the Point in the corresponding area with finger-press method, insert the filiform needle, which is #30 in diameter and 1. 0—1. 5 cun in length, for 0. 8 cun in depth. The insertion should be taken closely to the bone periosteum and along the radial aspect proximal to the palm border of the second Metacarpal bone. Change the direction of the needle tip until a strong needling sensation is found. It is possible to use the twirking and needle-retaining methods when this therapy is conducted. During the retention of the needle, manipulation should be done with intervals ranging from 5 to 10 minutes to retain the needling sensation. Oblique or perpendicular insertion can also be used.

图书在版编目(CIP)数据

现代针灸全书:技法篇/刘公望主编 . - 北京:华夏出版社,1998.10

ISBN 7 - 5080 - 1597 - 5

Ⅰ.现… Ⅱ.刘… Ⅲ.针灸疗法 Ⅳ.R245

中国版本图书馆 CIP 数据核字(98)第 28773 号

华 夏 出 版 社 出 版 发 行

(北京东直门外香河园北里 4 号　邮编:100028)

新 华 书 店 经 销

北 京 房 山 先 锋 印 刷 厂 印 刷

787×1092　1/16开本　12.25印张　378千字

1998 年 10 月北京第 1 版　　1998 年 10 月北京第 1 次印刷

印数 1 - 3000 册

定价:100.00 元

本版图书凡印刷、装订错误,可及时向我社发行部调换